58029

Psi 3

BAL: A+1

53-39

305244373V

An Atlas of
DEPRESSION

THE ENCYCLOPEDIA OF VISUAL MEDICINE SERIES

An Atlas of
DEPRESSION

David S. Baldwin

and

Jon Birtwistle
University of Southampton
Southampton, UK

The Parthenon Publishing Group
International Publishers in Medicine, Science & Technology

A CRC PRESS COMPANY
BOCA RATON   LONDON   NEW YORK   WASHINGTON, D.C.

Library of Congress Cataloging-in-Publication Data
Baldwin, David S.,
  An atlas of depression / David Baldwin and Jon Birtwistle.
  p. ; cm. -- (The encyclopedia of visual medicine series)
  Includes bibliographical references and index.
  ISBN 1-85070-942-4 (alk. paper)
  1. Depression, Mental--Atlases. I. Birtwistle, Jon. II. Title. III.
    Series.
  [DNLM: 1. Depressive Disorders--Atlases. 2. Anxiety
    Disorders--Atlases. WM 17 B181a 2002]
  RC537 .B337 2002
  616.85'27--dc21   2001056028

British Library Cataloguing in Publication Data
Baldwin, David, MB.
  An atlas of depression. - (The encyclopedia of visual medicine
  series)
  1.Depression, Mental
  I.Title II.Birtwistle, Jon
  616.8'527

  ISBN 1-85070-942-4

Published in the USA by
The Parthenon Publishing Group
345 Park Avenue South, 10th Floor
New York, NY 10010, USA

Published in the UK and Europe by
The Parthenon Publishing Group
23–25 Blades Court, Deodar Road
London, SW15 2NU, UK

Copyright © 2002 The Parthenon Publishing Group

Printed and bound by T.G. Hostench S.A., Spain

Contents

Preface

Depression is one of the most common forms of mental disorder in the general population. It has a lifetime prevalence as high as 15%, is associated with substantial morbidity and mortality, and imposes a substantial burden in developing and developed countries. According to recent data, unipolar major depression is the fifth leading cause of worldwide disability, accounting for around 4% of the world's total burden of disease.

Despite this, it is an obscure illness: people keep their depression secret; doctors choose not to recognize it; the cause is unknown; treatment is viewed with suspicion; and other conditions are given higher priority. Why is this?

No one likes to disclose problems that may be regarded as 'weakness' by others. People worry about the implications of disclosure on employment and insurance. Many are fearful of treatment, laboring under misapprehensions and misinformation promulgated by sensationalist and irresponsible journalists. Some doctors anticipate being overwhelmed by problems if they make the diagnosis of depression and choose to look aside. Mental health professionals are discouraged from the long-term treatment of people who may be regarded as having only 'minor' problems by purchasers of healthcare.

But the treatment of depression can be so rewarding. It is not difficult to recognize depression, providing the right questions are asked in the correct manner. Further assessment of recognized cases need not be excessively time-consuming. Doctors and patients can choose from a range of effective and acceptable treatments. People get better. Doctors feel satisfied. The burden of depression lifts.

This book aims to provide an introduction to the subject of depression. It is not a definitive textbook, but most aspects of the illness are covered in detail. Some aspects of the book reflect our personal clinical and research interests, but we hope the book retains sufficient balance in describing this common and debilitating disorder.

We would like the atlas to remain placed firmly on your desktop. The text should answer many of your queries about depression. The illustrations should also be helpful when describing causes and treatments during consultations with patients. Use it as you will. If it improves outcomes in just a few of your patients, it has done its job.

David S. Baldwin and Jon Birtwistle
January 2002

Section I   A Review of Depression

CHAPTER 1

Introduction

The affective or 'mood' disorders are a group of related conditions including the depressive disorders, mania and hypomania, in which the primary disturbance is thought to be one of mood or affect. The separation of the anxiety disorders from the depressive disorders into distinct diagnostic groups is the subject of some controversy. Anxiety and depressive syndromes show extensive overlap (comorbidity) in community, primary and secondary care settings (Figure 1.1), and a review by Piccinelli[1] concluded that there are no clear boundaries between major depression and generalized anxiety disorder. Therefore it is important that any discussion of depression must also include consideration of anxiety.

The key features of the depressive disorders are:

- low mood;
- reduced energy; and
- loss of interest or enjoyment.

Other common symptoms include poor concentration, reduced self-confidence, guilty thoughts, pessimism, ideas of self-harm or suicide, disturbed sleep and altered appetite[2] (see Figure 1.2).

Depression is a common disorder with serious personal, interpersonal and societal consequences, affecting about 15% of the general population and accounting for approximately 10% of consultations in primary care[3]. Women are twice as likely to suffer from depression, and symptoms generally increase with age. Recent studies suggest a rising incidence of depression in younger age groups, particularly young men, which may be linked to the relative rise in suicide rates. Whilst depressive symptoms are probably more frequent in the socially excluded and economically disadvantaged, depressive illness can affect people from all sections of society.

At a personal level depression causes significant psychologic distress, reduces quality of life and increases the mortality from cardiovascular disease, accidents and suicide, which is the cause of death in approximately 10% of patients with a severe recurrent depressive disorder. It can contribute to marital and family breakdown, and in depressed mothers may delay the development of their children. In addition there is a direct economic burden on society from health and social care costs, and indirectly through lost working days and the costs of premature mortality (see Table 1).

Table 1 The costs of depression in the UK[4]

Direct costs per annum	£300 million
Approximate cost of treated episode	£400
Indirect costs	£3 billion per annum
Working days lost	155 million per annum

Surveys of the general population in the UK reveal widespread negative public attitudes to depression. In a 1991 survey of the public conducted on behalf of the United Kingdom Defeat Depression Campaign[5], only 16% believed people with depression should be treated with antidepressants, while 90% thought counseling should be used, which has disputed efficacy in the treatment of depression. In addition, the vast majority (78%) of the sampled general population believed that antidepressant drugs are 'addictive', probably confusing them with benzodiazepine anxiolytics.

The overall management of people with depression is often far from ideal (see Figure 1.3). Stigma and discrimination make people who might be suffering from depression reluctant to seek treatment, and the recognition of depression by doctors and other health professionals is often poor. When these factors are taken together, depression can clearly be seen to constitute a major public health issue (see Table 2).

Table 2 Criteria for a condition to be a public health issue

- common
- severe
- marked associated impairment
- effective treatments
- acceptable treatments
- significant public concern

REFERENCES

1. Piccinelli M. Comorbidity of depression and generalised anxiety: is there any distinct boundary? *Curr Opin Psychiatry* 1998;11:57–60

2. World Health Organization. *The ICD-10 Classification of Mental and Behavioural Disorders*. Clinical descriptions and diagnosis guidelines. Geneva : WHO, 1992

3. Ormel J, Tiemens B. Depression in primary care. In: Honig A, van Praag HM, eds. *Depression: Neurobiological, Psychopathological and Therapeutic Advances*. Chichester, UK: John Wiley, 1997

4. Chisholm D. The economic consequences of depression. In: Dawson A, Tylee A, eds. *Depression: social and economic time-bomb*. London: BMJ Books, 2001:121–9

5. MORI Poll. *Defeat Depression Campaign*. London, MORI, 1992

BIBLIOGRAPHY

Wells KB, Stewart A, Hays RD, *et al*. The functioning and well-being of depressed patients. Results from the Medical Outcomes Study. *JAMA* 1989;262:914–19

CHAPTER 2

Epidemiology

INTRODUCTION

The introduction of the American Psychiatric Association Diagnostic and Statistical Manual (DSM-III in 1980 and DSM-IV in 1994) and the World Health Organization International Classification of Diseases (ICD-10 in 1992) has resulted in development of operational criteria for mental and behavioral disorders (see Figures 2.1 and 2.2). This in turn has made it possible to perform large cross-sectional epidemiologic surveys to compare prevalence rates across various cultures and communities, and between primary and secondary care settings.

INCIDENCE AND PREVALENCE

The frequency of a condition is generally reported in terms of 'incidence' and 'prevalence'. The incidence is the rate at which new cases occur in a population during a specified period. If the population at risk is constant then:

$$I = N/(P \times T)$$

(I, incidence; N, number of new cases; P, population at risk; T, time during which cases were ascertained)

By contrast, the prevalence of a disease is the proportion of a population that are cases at a point in time. When a disorder occurs intermittently, a single assessment in time gives a 'point' prevalence, which could underestimate the frequency of the condition. A better measure is one that uses a stated time period (e.g. 1 month, 6 months, 12 months or a lifetime) and assesses the frequency of cases within that time.

'CASENESS'

To be included in the disease count a person must be diagnosed as being a 'case'. Diagnosis requires a clear definition of the condition, in the form of operational criteria against which to compare a patient's symptoms (such as those included in the DSM-IV and ICD-10 criteria). Some medical conditions show a clear dichotomy between 'case' and 'non-case' (e.g. Down syndrome), but most fall somewhere along a continuum of severity (see Figure 2.3). Much of psychiatric diagnosis is at this level, ranging in intensity from minimal subthreshold symptoms to extreme and disabling symptoms.

Epidemiologic research is hindered by a number of methodologic problems, which should be considered when comparing incidence and prevalence rates. The test–retest reliability can be poor, as the recollection of affect is often inaccurate and memory and concentration problems are features of most mental disorders. The assessment instruments developed within the construct of the diagnostic categories of DSM and ICD may lack sensitivity in primary care and community settings, where psychiatric problems are frequently less severe and persistent and many cases are subthreshold, i.e. do not fulfil the criteria for a full diagnosis.

GENDER

Approximately 15% of the general population report depressive symptoms, with 10% of primary care consultations being due to depressive disorders[1]. Most cross-cultural community surveys have found major depressive disorder to be about twice as prevalent in women as in men, the lifetime prevalence being approximately 20% compared to 10%, respectively[2]. There is some evidence that women develop more complex and severe clinical pictures, and probably a more troublesome course[3]. The reason for this gender difference is unclear, although greater childcare responsibilities and fewer opportunities for paid employment may be important factors. However, men are known to report fewer problems, and seek help for emotional problems less frequently.

AGE

In the elderly there appears to be a 'leveling out' of the gender difference for major depression, although the overall prevalence of depressive symptoms appears to increase with age (see Figure 2.4). Several studies suggest a rising incidence of depression in younger age groups, particularly in young men, which may be linked to the relative rise in suicide rates in this age group when compared to the declining rates in the general population[4]. Major depression in childhood is no longer considered rare, the point prevalence in children lying in the range 0.5–2.5%[5]. Depression is notably more common in adolescents than in younger children, having an average period prevalence of around 3–4%[6].

COMORBIDITY

Depression and anxiety usually occur together, both in community and clinical samples. Approximately two-thirds of those with a lifetime history of major depression have a lifetime history of another psychiatric disorder, and an even higher proportion of those with anxiety have multiple previous disorders. Some of the 'comorbidity' of anxiety and depression is artifactual, due to the categorical approach to psychiatric diagnosis.

The use of a more 'dimensional' approach, in which the severity of individual symptoms and signs is described – rather than the current categorical approach, which involves counting symptoms – would reduce this apparent comorbidity. Patients with significant coexisting depressive and anxiety symptoms have a poorer prognosis with greater impairment, greater persistence of symptoms, increased use of health service resources and an increased risk of suicidal behavior.

REFERENCES

1. Ormel J, Tiemens B. Depression in primary care. In Honig A, van Praag HM, eds. *Depression: Neurobiological, Psychopathological and Therapeutic Advances*. Chichester, UK: John Wiley, 1997

2. Patel V. Cultural factors and international epidemiology. *Br Med Bull* 2001;57:33–45

3. Angst J. Epidemiology of depression. In Honig A, van Praag HM, eds. *Depression: Neurobiological, Psychopathological and Therapeutic Advances*. Chichester, UK: John Wiley, 1997

4. Fombonne E. True trends in affective disorders. In: Cohen P, Slomkoski C, Robins LN, eds. *Historical and Geographical Influences on Psychopathology*. New Jersey: Laurence Erlbaum, 1999:115–39

5. Harrington R. Epidemiology. In: Harrington R, ed. *Depressive Disorder in Childhood Adolescence*. Chichester, UK: John Wiley, 1993

6. Fombonne E. The epidemiology of child and adolescent depression psychiatric disorders: recent developments and issues. *Epidemiol Psychiatric Soc* 1998;7:161–6

CHAPTER 3

Recognition of depression

INTRODUCTION

In primary care the recognition of depression is often less than ideal. For example, 50% of people with major depression, identified by independent screening in GP waiting rooms, are not recognized as depressed by the doctor[1]. The recognition of depression is particularly difficult in certain patient groups such as the physically ill.

POSSIBLE REASON FOR LACK OF RECOGNITION

There may be a number of possible reasons for a lack of recognition of depression within primary care (see Figure 3.1). Generally these can be summarized as follows:

- patients ignore depression in themselves;

- fear of the stigma of mental illness;

- worry about side effects of medication;

- misdiagnosis of somatic complaints;

- overlooking of depression in those known to have a physical illness; and

- blaming depression on circumstances, regarding it as 'understandable'.

Unfortunately those patients who go unrecognized and untreated may have poorer short-term outcomes on measures of low mood, reduced energy and irritability. However, recent research suggests that disclosure of depression in 'unrecognized' patients has little effect on overall outcome.

There are a number of key interview skills and cues that have been identified as crucial to the recognition of depression (see Figures 3.2 and 3.3).

IS DEPRESSION MORE COMMON TODAY?

There is some evidence that the incidence of depression may have increased in younger cohorts. A long-term follow-up study in Sweden (the Lundby Study)[2] found a marked increase in incidence rates in the 1960s and 1970s, and a ten-fold increase in the incidence for men aged 20–39 years, for the period of 1957–1972 compared to 1947–1957, although this may be due to a limited amount of data before the 1960s, against which to make a valid comparison. Although there have been several studies that indicate a recent rise in the incidence and prevalence of depression, this remains fairly controversial due to methodologic problems in data collection, particularly the recall bias for remembering symptoms from more recent years.

REFERENCES

1. Goldberg DP, Huxley P. *Mental illness in the community. The pathway to psychiatric care.* London: Tavistock, 1980

2. Hagnell O, Lanke J, Rorsman B, Ojesjo L. Are we entering an age of melancholy? Depressive illnesses in a prospective epidemiological study over 25 years: the Lundby Study, Sweden. *Psychol Med* 1982;12:279–89

CHAPTER 4

Descriptions of the depressive disorders

INTRODUCTION

The ICD-10 and DSM-IV have largely similar approaches to the classification of the depressive disorders (see Figures 2.1 and 2.2), with a depressive episode (ICD-10) and a major depressive episode (DSM-IV) being the pivotal form of depressive illness, about which other depressive disorders are described. However, in primary care, many depressed patients present with depressive symptoms that do not fulfil the accepted diagnostic criteria for major depression or depressive episode, because the depressive syndrome is too mild, too short, too long or without social consequences. By contrast patients in secondary care inpatient settings are rather unrepresentative of the total sample of patients, psychiatrists being likely to see the most severely ill and those patients with 'comorbid' (coexisting) disorders.

The most recent classificatory schemes include a number of other depressive disorders, in an attempt to describe important groups of patients, who otherwise could not be allocated a diagnosis. For example, both the DSM-IV classification and the ICD-10 system include dysthymia (a chronic mild depressive disorder), and the ICD-10 also incorporates recurrent brief depressive disorder (RBD) within the group of mood disorders.

UNIPOLAR AND BIPOLAR DEPRESSION

When a person develops an episode of mania they are conventionally identified as suffering from bipolar disorder, but those patients with depressive episodes only are diagnosed as having unipolar depression. This differentiation is useful from a clinical perspective, as differing treatment approaches are required for these disorders (see Figure 4.1). The person who is in a manic phase of the bipolar disorder will usually require 'anti-manic' treatment, and treatment of any future depressive episodes must be carefully undertaken, so as not to precipitate a further manic episode.

Most patients experience multiple depressive episodes over their lifetime, the episodes varying in length, severity and impairment, and in the response to treatment. Approximately 15% of consultations in general practice are due to 'recurrent unipolar depression'[1]. Anxiety symptoms are a common feature in many people with depression and may be so prominent that they 'mask' the underlying depressive symptoms, which are found only after direct questioning.

MAJOR DEPRESSIVE EPISODE

The two key features of major depression are depressed mood and loss of interest or pleasure.

The prevailing mood is one of persistent misery, which does not respond to good news. This is often accompanied by a lack of enthusiasm for previously enjoyable activities or hobbies. Figure 2.2 shows the DSM-IV diagnostic criteria for major depressive episode.

The lifetime prevalence rates for major depressive disorder have been estimated to range between 12% and 17%. However, there is a wide variation in the reported prevalence rates for major depression (see Figure 4.2). Table 1 shows the lifetime prevalence rates found across a variety of locations[27]. The lowest rates were 0.9% in Taiwan, and the highest 24% in Oregon (USA). European rates are closer to those of Oregon, e.g. 15.7% in Basel[18,19], 16% in Zurich[27] and 16.4% in Paris[21]. A key factor in identifying rates of major depression is the sensitivity of the questionnaire instrument. The Composite International Diagnostic Schedule (CIDI) is probably a more sensitive instrument than the Diagnostic Interview Schedule (DIS), which generally produces lower rates.

Table I Lifetime prevalence rates of major depressive disorder. CIDI, Composite International Diagnostic Schedule; DIS, Diagnostic Interview Schedule; DSM-III-R, Diagnostic and Statistic Manual III revised; HDS (DPA), Diagnostic and statistic Manual I revised; NCS, National Comorbidity Survey; SADS-L, schedule for affective disorders and schizophrenia; SADS-RDC, schedule for affective disorders and schizophrenia – research diagnostic criteria. Adapted with permission from Angst J. *The Prevalence of Depression in Antidepressant Therapy at the Dawn of the Third Millennium.* Briley M, Montgomery S, eds. London: Dunitz, 1998:198

Location	Reference	Instrument	n	Male	Female	Male + Female
Taiwan (metropolis)	2	DIS	5005	0.7	1.0+	0.9
Taiwan (small township)	3	DIS	3004	0.9	2.5+	1.7
Hong Kong	4	DIS	7229	1.3	2.4	–
Korea	5	DIS	3134	2.4	4.1	3.3
Korea (rural)	6	DIS	2995	2.9	4.1	3.5
Puerto Rico	7	DIS	1513	3.5	5.5	4.6
Iceland	8	DIS/DSM-III	862	2.9	7.8	5.3
ECA, USA	9	DIS		5.2	10.2	4.9
New Haven, USA	9	DIS	5063	–	–	5.9
Baltimore, USA	9	DIS	3560	–	–	3.0
St Louis, USA	9	DIS	3200	–	–	4.5
Durham, USA	9	DIS	4101	–	–	3.5
Los Angeles, USA	9	DIS	3436	–	–	5.6
Mainz, Germany	10	SADS-L	80	–	–	7.7
National Survey, USA	11					8.4
Edmonton, Canada	12	DIS	3258	5.9	11.4	8.6
Munich, Germany	13	DIS	483	–	–	9.0
Boston, USA	14	DIS DSM-III-R	386	5.1	13.7	9.4
Sardinia	15	CIDI	552	11.6	14.8	13.3
Christchurch, New Zealand	16	DIS	1498	8.8	16.3	12.6
St Louis, USA	17	DIS	298	12.8	23.8	14.8
Basel, Switzerland	18,19	CIDI	470	11.0	19.5	15.7
Stirling County, Canada	20	HDS (DPA)	1003			16.0
Paris	21	DIS/CIDI	1787	10.7	22.4	16.4
NCS, USA	22,23	CIDI	8098	F	F	17.1
New Haven, USA	24	SADS-RDC		12.3	25.8	18.0
Oregon (T$_1$)	25	SADS-L	1508	11.6	24.8	18.5
Oregon (T$_2$)	25			15.2	31.6	24.0
Iceland	26	DIS	862	2.0	7.8	–

DYSTHYMIA (DYSTHYMIC DISORDER)

Dysthymia was first introduced into the group of affective disorders in the DSM-III classification in 1980. It overlaps substantially with major depression, the main differentiation being that dysthymia is a chronic depressive disorder with milder symptoms. The chronic features of dysthymia fluctuate in severity, and most sufferers will develop supervening comorbid major depressive episodes (sometimes termed 'double depression'). See Figure 4.3 for a summary of the DSM-IV criteria.

Estimates of lifetime prevalence of dysthymia are probably unreliable. A review by Angst[28] revealed a lifetime prevalence ranging from 1.1% to 20.6%. Accurate diagnosis is often difficult and the reliability low, since it

is largely dependent on the accurate recall of symptoms spanning 2 years, which may be many years in the patient's past. The female:male ratio is approximately 2:1, and dysthymia appears more common in the elderly than in younger people. In one study of a Finnish cohort of elderly subjects the prevalence was 12%[29].

RECURRENT BRIEF DEPRESSION

Community studies, predominantly of young adults, indicate that many people receiving treatment for depression do not fulfil the diagnostic criteria for major depression[30]. Some experience shorter episodes of depression, i.e. lasting less than 2 weeks. For some the depressive episodes recur at least monthly, and are brief, but usually severe, with significant social and occupational impairment and sometimes associated with suicidal behavior. Figure 4.4 show the 'Zurich criteria' for recurrent brief depression (RBD). Broadly similar descriptions are now included within ICD-10 and Appendix B of DSM-IV.

Although RBD appears to be common in the community there has been relatively little research into the epidemiology of the condition. One-year prevalence rates vary between 4% and 8%[28]; 14.6% of the population in the Zurich study had fulfilled criteria for RBD by the age of 35 years. The WHO primary care study found a point prevalence of 5.2% for 'pure' RBD, together with a rate of 4.8% for RBD associated with other depressive disorders[31].

MIXED ANXIETY AND DEPRESSIVE DISORDER

The ICD-10 includes a category of mixed anxiety and depressive disorder (MADD), to be recorded when symptoms of both anxiety and depression are present, but neither set of symptoms, considered separately, is sufficiently severe to justify a diagnosis. The appendix of the DSM-IV contains a broadly similar description, but neither ICD-10 nor DSM-IV have specified criteria. The recent UK Office of Population Censuses and Surveys (OPCS) Survey of Psychiatric Morbidity found a point prevalence for MADD (using ICD-10 diagnostic criteria) of 7.7%, compared to a point prevalence of only 2.1%, for depressive episodes[32], rates in women being almost double those in men (9.9% versus 5.4%, respectively). The course and treatment outcome of MADD are largely unknown, but the disorder is likely to be of particular relevance in primary care settings.

SEASONAL AFFECTIVE DISORDER

Seasonal affective disorder (SAD) was described originally by Rosenthal and colleagues in 1984[33], and can be diagnosed using either ICD-10 or DSM-IV criteria. DSM-IV describes SAD as being a mood disorder with an established seasonal pattern (see Figure 4.5). Seasonal variations in mood are well established and have been commented on by numerous sources ranging from Aretaeus and Hippocrates, to Shakespeare in *The Winter's Tale*: "a sad tale's best for winter". Although the concept of 'seasonal affective disorder' has gained a degree of recognition in both the ICD-10 and DSM-IV

classifications, there is little epidemiologic support for its being considered a separate depressive disorder. Depression occurring in the darker seasons of autumn and winter has been dubbed 'winter blues' and is believed by some to be due to the lack of sunlight, particularly in the northern hemisphere. But there is little agreement on which seasons have the peak incidences of depressed mood, as it can occur in autumn, winter, spring and even late summer! The current criteria for SAD state that there should be at least three episodes of mood disturbance in three separate years, of which two or more years are consecutive. As follow-up studies indicate that many patients with 'SAD' develop significant non-seasonal depressive episodes, the criteria stipulate that seasonal episodes should outnumber non-seasonal episodes by more than 3:1.

POSTPARTUM DEPRESSION

Approximately 29% of women after childbirth experience some mild decline in mood and/or increased anxiety, thought mainly to be due to psychosocial changes associated with motherhood[34]. Most do not require treatment. However, postpartum depression affects 14% of women. The features generally fit the DSM-IV criteria for major depression and the diagnosis is given when the onset is within 4 weeks postpartum, as defined in the 'postpartum onset specifier'. Anxiety is often a prominent feature with high levels of anxiety, particularly obsessional ruminations about the health of the infant.

BIPOLAR AFFECTIVE DISORDER (MANIC-DEPRESSIVE PSYCHOSIS)

Community surveys in industrialized countries estimate a 1% lifetime risk for bipolar disorder and a 5% risk for the bipolar spectrum[35]. In 1990, bipolar disorder was estimated to be the sixth leading cause of worldwide disability in people between the ages of 15 and 44 years (see Figure 4.6)[36]. The mean age of onset is 21 years, which is earlier than for major depression. Both sexes are affected equally, although women tend to have proportionately more depressive episodes. The cyclical pattern of mania and depression was previously called 'manic-depressive psychosis'. The current term of bipolar affective disorder or bipolar illness is more appropriate, as many patients with marked disturbance of affect do not ever experience psychotic phenomena, such as delusions or hallucinations.

Emotional highs or elation are normal responses to happy events or good fortune. However, elation or 'mania', which seems to occur without any obvious cause, or appears excessive or too prolonged, may be a symptom or sign of several psychiatric syndromes, including manic episodes, acute schizophrenic episodes and certain drug-induced states (see Figure 4.7). Mania-like episodes can also occur as a result of some medical conditions (e.g. hyperthyroidism), prescribed medication, nonprescribed psychoactive substances (e.g. amphetamines, cocaine, caffeine) or antidepressant treatments (antidepressant drugs, electroconvulsive therapy, light therapy). Such manic-like episodes do not fulfil the diagnostic criteria for a manic episode. Figure 4.8 shows the DSM-IV criteria for mania.

There are four key diagnostic categories in DSM-IV:

- bipolar I – at least one manic episode with or without a depressive episode;

- bipolar II – one hypomanic episode and at least one depressive episode;

- cyclothymia – long-term depressive and hypomanic symptoms but no episodes of major depression, hypomania or mania; and

- mixed episode – criteria are met for both a manic episode and for major depression nearly every day for at least a 1-week period.

People experiencing manic episodes often appear euphoric with abundant energy and increased activity and decreased need for sleep, which is usually accompanied by an exaggerated sense of subjective well-being. This is generally reflected in excessive talking (pressure of speech), grandiose ideas and unrealistic plans. However, many also feel irritable and exasperated, and the euphoric mood is sometimes tinged with sadness. Judgement is typically impaired; this can lead to financial or sexual indiscretions that may ruin personal and family life. Insight into the changes in mood, activity and interpersonal relationships is usually reduced. The mean duration of mania is 2–3 months.

Manic episodes rarely occur in isolation: more characteristically, episodes recur irregularly, becoming interspersed with depressive episodes, which may become relatively more frequent as time passes. Episodes of illness tend to cluster at particular times in a patient's life, for example when relationships are ending or when employment is changed.

DEPRESSION AND ANXIETY AFTER BEREAVEMENT

One of the main consequences of bereavement is psychologic distress, particularly sadness and depression. Other features include anxiety, insomnia, somatic symptoms (somatization) and hallucinations. In western culture, the expression of sadness following bereavement is expected and its absence seen as pathologic. In addition to bereavement, a sense of grief can be experienced from other major losses, such as a terminal diagnosis, losing a job, a marriage that fails, amputation or radical surgery. Figures 4.9 and 4.10 show typical physical and psychologic symptoms experienced during 'normal grief'.

Bereavement can also have a negative impact on health. There is an increased risk of mortality particularly within the first 6 months after bereavement[37–40]. There is also evidence of an increased vulnerability to physical illness and mortality during the first 2 years of bereavement, with men at higher risk than women. Some bereaved people develop health-impairing behaviors such as increased substance use[41], typically alcohol, tobacco and psychotropic medication[42], which can have negative consequences for mental and physical health.

Marital status has an important influence on the rates of depressive disorders both in the community and inpatients and, in general, those who are widowed or divorced have a greater risk of depression than those married or single. Bebbington[43] analyzed data from English national statistics to assess the association between sex, marital status and first admission to psychiatric hospital. First admission rates (1982–1985) were estimated per 100 000 for populations over the age of 15 using ICD-9 as the diagnostic criteria. Admission rates for all depressive disorders were higher in widowed and divorced patients irrespective of gender. When all affective disorders were taken together, those widowed had the highest incidence.

Bereavement also increases the risk of mental health problems, particularly depression and anxiety[44–46]. Symptoms of anxiety and depression are common during the first months of bereavement and normal grief reactions persists for 2–6 months, but usually improve without specific interventions.

However, there are particular methodologic concerns with much of the earlier bereavement research including small samples, recruitment methods leading to biased samples, an overrepresentation of spousal bereavement, non-valid outcome measures and high rates of dropout at follow-up, but most well designed studies have produced consistent results. Symptoms of anxiety and depression generally peak during the first 6 months of bereavement and normally improve from the sixth month with the majority of people being comparable to their pre-bereavement state after the first year[44,47].

Zisook and Schuchter[44] measured the frequency of depressive syndromes at 2, 7 and 13 months after the death of a spouse and compared them to a married control group. In those bereaved, the percentage who met DSM-III-R criteria for depressive episodes was 24% at 2 months, 23% at 7 months and 16% at 13 months. The prevalence of depressive episodes in the control group was 4%. Factors that predicted depression at 13 months were younger age, history of major depression, still grieving at 2 months after the loss and being depressed at 2 and/or 7 months after the death.

Being a younger widow appears to be a risk factor for prolonged depressive reaction and increased risk of other mental health problems. Those bereaved before 65 years of age appear to be at greater risk of psychiatric problems. In a study of the medical records of 44 unselected widows, psychiatric symptoms (depression and anxiety) were found to predominate in the younger bereaved (< 65 years), while physical symptoms predominated in the older bereaved (> 65 years)[48]. Widows over 65 years appear to demonstrate a qualitatively different reaction to bereavement. However, about one-third of widowed elderly people meet DSM-III-R criteria for a major depressive episode 1 month after the loss and one-quarter 2–7 months after the loss[49,50].

Mendes-de-Leon and colleagues[45] carried out a prospective study of 1046 elderly people married at baseline of whom 139 were widowed during the 3-year follow-up. Depression before and after the bereavement was measured using the Center for Epidemiological Studies–Depression scale (CES-D). Those who had been bereaved for 6 months or less had a 75% increase in depressive symptoms.

Most returned to baseline levels by the second year of bereavement. However, young-old widows (defined as 65–74 years old) appeared to differ in the reaction to bereavement and showed increased levels of depressive symptoms into the second and third years of bereave-

ment. This was a risk factor for developing chronic depression following bereavement.

For bereaved adults, having friends or neighbors to turn to seems to be a protective factor against emotional problems such as depression, loneliness and worry. In one prospective study by Goldberg and colleagues[51], a cohort of 1144 married women were interviewed in 1979 about their health and social networks. Within 2.5 years 150 had become widows. Of those 128, aged between 65 and 78 years were interviewed 6 months after bereavement. Twenty-two percent stated that they had required counseling for an emotional problem. Factors associated with emotional difficulties included recent disability, having few friends and not feeling close to one's children.

Parkes[52] suggests that anxiety is the most common response to bereavement. In the opening paragraph of *A Grief Observed*, C.S. Lewis describes the overwhelming feelings of grief he experienced after the death of his wife. "No one ever told me that grief felt so much like fear. I am not afraid, but the sensation is like being afraid. The same fluttering in the stomach, the same restlessness, the yawning. I keep on swallowing"[53].

Jacobs and colleagues[46] assessed 102 widowed people aged 21–65; 48 were assessed at 6 months and 54 at 12 months after bereavement. Overall 44.4% reported at least one type of anxiety during the second half of the year, 25% in the first 6 months. The risk of panic disorder (PD) and generalized anxiety disorder (GAD) in the second 6-month period of the year was about double the rate in the first 6 months of bereavement. The predictors of PD were a history of PD, while the predictors for GAD were younger age, history of anxiety disorders and history of depression.

There were also associations with depression; 55.6% (20 of 36) who had anxiety disorder also reported a depressive syndrome. All of those with GAD also met the criteria for major depression and 60% of those with PD also met the criteria for depression. Conversely 82.5% of participants with a depressive disorder also met the criteria for at least one anxiety disorder. When depression was diagnosed it was always associated with the diagnosis of GAD.

REFERENCES

1. Üstün TB, Sartorius. *Mental Illness in General Health Care.* Chichester, UK: John Wiley, 1995

2. Hwu EK, Hwu HG, Cheng LY, *et al.* Lifetime prevalence of mental disorders in a Chinese metropolis and 2 townships. In: *Proceedings, International Symposium in Psychiatric Epidemiology.* Taipei City, 1985

3. Hwu HG, Yeh EK, Chang LY. Prevalence of psychiatric disorders in Taiwan defined by the Chinese Diagnostic Interview Schedule. *Acta Psychiatr Scand* 1989;79:136–47

4. Chen CN, Wong J, Lee N, *et al.* The Shatin community mental health survey in Hong Kong. II. Major findings. *Arch Gen Psychiatry* 1993;50:125–33

5. Lee CK, Kwak YS, Yamamoto J, *et al.* Psychiatric epidemiology in Korea. Part I: gender and age differences in Seoul. *J Nerv Ment Dis* 1990;178:242–6

6. Lee CK, Kwak YS, Yamamoto J, *et al.* Psychiatric epidemiology in Korea. Part II: urban and rural differences. *J Nerv Ment Dis* 1990;178:247–52

7. Canino GJ, Bird HR, Shrout PE, *et al.* The prevalence of specific psychiatric disorders in Puerto Rico. *Arch Gen Psychiatry* 1987;44:727–35

8. Stefànsson JG, Lindal E, Björnsson JK, *et al.* Lifetime prevalence of specific mental disorders among people born in Iceland. *Acta Psychiatr Scand* 1991; 84:142–9

9. Weissman MM, Bruce LM, Leaf PJ, *et al.* Affective disorders. In: Robins LN, Regier DA, eds. *Psychiatric Disorders in America. The Epidemiologic Catchment Area Study.* New York: The Free Press, 1990:53–80

10. Heun R, Maier W. The distinction of bipolar II disorder from bipolar I and recurrent unipolar depression: results of a controlled family study. *Acta Psychiatr Scand* 1993;87:279–84

11. Elliot D, Huizinger D, Morse BJ. The dynamics of deviant behaviour. A National Survey: Progress Report. Boulder, CO: Behavioral Research Institute, 1985

12. Bland RC, Orn H, Newman SC. Lifetime prevalence of psychiatric disorders in Edmonton. *Acta Psychiatr Scand* 1988;338 (suppl):24–32

13. Wittchen HU, von Zerssen D. *Verläufe behandelter und unbehandelter Depressionen und Angstsörungen. Eine Klinisch-psychiatrische und epidemiologische Verlaufs-untersuchung.* Berlin: Springer, 1987

14. Reinherz HZ, Giaconia RM, Lefkowitz ES, Pakiz B, Frost AK. Prevalence of psychiatric disorders in a community population of older adolescents. *J Am Acad Child Adolesc Psychiatry* 1993;32:369–77

15. Carta MG, Carpiniello B, Porcedda R. Lifetime prevalence of major depression and dysthymia: results of a community survey in Sardinia. *Eur Neuropsychopharmacol* 1995; suppl:103–7

16. Wells KB, Stewart A, Hays RD, *et al.* The functioning and well-being of depressed patients. Results from the medical outcomes study. *JAMA* 1989;262:914–19

17. Oliver JM, Simmons ME. Affective disorders and depression as measured by the Diagnostic Interview Schedule and the Beck Depression Inventory in an unselected adult population. *J Clin Psychol* 1985;41:469–76

18. Wacker HR. *Angst und Depression. Eine Epidemiologische Untersuchung.* Bern, Switzerland: Hans Huber, 1985

19. Wacker HR, Müllejahns R, Klein KH, *et al.* Identification of cases of anxiety disorders and affective disorders in the community according to ICD-10 and DSM-III-R by using the Composite International Diagnostic Interview (CIDI). *Int J Meth Psychiatr Res* 1992;2:91–100

20. Murphy JM. Continuities in community-based psychiatric epidemiology. *Arch Gen Psychiatry* 1980;37:1215–23

21. Lepine JP. Comorbidity of anxiety and depression: epidemiologic perspectives [in French]. *Encephale* 1994;20:683–92

22. Kessler RC, McGonagle KA, Nelson CB, *et al.* Sex and depression in the National Comorbidity Survey. II: Cohort effects. *J Affect Disord* 1994;30:15–26

23. Blazer DG, Kessler RC, McGonagle KA, Swartz MS. The prevalence and distribution of major depression in a national community sample: the National Comorbidity Survey. *Am J Psychiatry* 1994;151:979–86

24. Weissman MM, Myers JK. Affective disorders in a US urban community. The use of research diagnostic criteria in an epidemiological survey. *Arch Gen Psychiatry* 1978;35:1304–11

25. Lewinsohn PM, Hops H, Roberts RE, Seeley JR, Andrews JA. Adolescent psychopathology: I. Prevalence and incidence of depression and other DSM-III-R disorders in high school students. *J Abnorm Psychol* 1993;102:133–44

26. Lindal E, Stefànsson JG. The frequency of depressive symptoms in a general population with reference to DSM-III. *Int J Soc Psychiatry* 1991;37:233–41

27. Angst J. Epidemiology of depression. In: Honig A, van Praag HM, eds. *Depression: Neurobiological, Psychopathological and Therapeutic Advances.* Chichester, UK: John Wiley, 1997

28. Angst J. The epidemiology of dysthymia. *Perspect Depr* 1995;3:1–5

29. Pahkala K, Kesti E, Kongas-Saviaro P, Laippala P, Kivela SL. Prevalence of depression in an aged population in Finland. *Soc Psychaitry Psychiatr Epidemiol* 1995:30:99–106

30. Angst J, Merikangas K, Scheidegger P, Wicki W. Recurrent brief depression: a new subtype of affective disorder. *J Affect Disord* 1990;19:87–98

31. Weiller E, Boyer P, Lepine JP, Lecrubier Y. Prevalence of recurrent brief depression in primary care. *Eur Arch Psychiatry Clin Neurosci* 1994;244:174–81

32. Meltzer H, The prevalence of psychiatric morbidity among adults living in private households. In: *OPCS Surveys of Psychiatric Morbidity in Great Britain*, Report 1. London: OPCS Social Survey Division, 1995

33. Rosenthal NE, Sack DA, Gillin JC, *et al.* Seasonal affective disorder: a description of the syndrome and preliminary findings with light therapy. *Arch General Psychiatry* 1984,41:72–80

34. Denerstein *et al.* Postpartum depression – risk factors. *J Psychosom Obstet Gynaecol* 1989;10 (suppl):53–65

35. Weissman MM, Bland RC, Canino GJ, *et al.* Cross-national epidemiology of major depression and bipolar disorder. *JAMA* 1996;276:293–9

36. Murray CJL, Lopez AD, eds. *The Global Burden of Disease: a Comprehensive Assessment of Mortality and Disability from Diseases, Injuries, and Risk Factors in 1990 and Projected to 2020.* Boston: Harvard University Press, 1996

37. Young M, Benjamin B, Wallis C. Mortality of widowers. *Lancet* 1963;2:454–6

38. Rees WD, Lutkins SG. Mortality of bereavement. *Br Med J* 1967;4:13–16

39. Martikainen P, Valkonen T. Mortality after death of a spouse in relation to duration of bereavement in Finland. *J Epidemiol Community Health* 1996;50:264–8

40. Lichtenstein P, Gatz M, Berg S. A twin study of mortality after spousal bereavement. *Psychol Med* 1998;28:635–43

41. Stroebe MS, Stroebe W. Who suffers more? Sex differences in health risks of the widowed. *Psychol Bull* 1983;93:279–301

42. Parkes CM, Brown RJ. Health after bereavement. A controlled study of young Boston widows and widowers. *Psychosom Med* 1972;34:449–61

43. Bebbington P. Marital status and depression: a study of English national admission statistics. *Acta Psychiatr Scand* 1987; 75: 640–50

44. Zisook S, Shuchter SR. Depression through the first year after the death of a spouse. *Am J Psychiatry* 1991;148:1346–52

45. Mendes-De-Leon CF, Kasl LS, Jacobs SA. Prospective study of widowhood and changes in symptoms of depression in a community sample of the elderly. *Psychol Med* 1994;24:613–24

46. Jacobs S, Hansen F, Kasl S, Ostfeld A, Berkman L, Kim K. Anxiety disorders during acute bereavement: risk and risk factors *J Clin Psychiatry* 1990;51:269–74

47. Bornstein PE, Clayton PJ, Halikas JA, Maurice WL, Robins E. The depression of widowhood after thirteen months. *Br J Psychiatry* 1973;122:561–6

48. Parkes CM. The effects of bereavement on physical and mental health: a study of the case records of widows. *Br Med J* 1964;2:274–9

49. Clayton PJ, Halikas JA, Maurice WL. The depression of widowhood. *Br J Psychiatry* 1972;120:71–8

50. Jacobs SC, Hansen FF, Berkman L, *et al.* Depressions of bereavement. *Compr Psychiatry* 1989;30:218–24

51. Goldberg EL, Comstock GW, Harlow SD. Emotional problems and widowhood. *J Gerontol* 1988;43:206–8

52. Parkes CM. *Bereavement, Studies of Grief in Adult Life.* London: Penguin Books, 1996

53. Lewis CS. *A Grief Observed.* London: Faber and Faber, 1961

CHAPTER 5

Clinical descriptions of the anxiety disorders

INTRODUCTION

Anxiety and depressive symptoms usually co-exist (see Figure 5.1). If each syndrome is relatively mild, patients may fulfil the criteria for mixed anxiety and depressive disorder. However, when symptoms are more severe, patients can be regarded as having coexisting or 'comorbid' anxiety and depressive disorders.

Human beings have an innate 'biological pre-preparedness' to respond with 'anxious' feelings to certain stimuli, such as threat of violence and fear of heights. The underlying evolutionary function is that of an 'alarm' mechanism (the 'fight or flight response') to prepare an individual for a physical response to perceived danger (see Figure 5.2). Not only do humans respond to their immediate environment but also they anticipate events and plan for the future. So the anticipation of the events at some future time (e.g. pre-exam nerves, visits to the dentist) can also initiate the alarm. Anxiety is a normal emotional response to a perceived threat or stressful events – it is usually short-lived and controllable. Table 1 shows the psychologic and physical symptoms of anxiety, most of which are attributable to autonomic arousal.

However, when the symptoms of anxiety are abnormally severe, unusually prolonged or occur in the absence of stressful circumstances and/or impair physical, social or occupational functioning, it can be viewed as a clinically significant disorder beyond the 'normal' emotional response. In reality anxiety is best viewed as being a continuum from mild personal distress to severe mental disorder. Approximately 5–7% of the general population experience clinically important anxiety, as do 25% or more of patients in medical settings at any one time. The National Comorbidity Survey in the United States suggest that the lifetime prevalence of anxiety disorders may be as high as 28.7%[1]. In practice the dis-

tinction between normal responses to threat and anxiety disorders may sometimes be difficult to make.

There are a number of medical conditions that produce anxiety symptoms, making diagnosis challenging and raising the risk of incorrect diagnosis and, in some cases, the non-detection of underling physical illness. Anxiety symptoms are a feature of caffeinism, alcohol and drug withdrawal, hyperthyroidism, hypoglycemia, paroxysmal tachycardia, complex partial seizures (temporal lobe epilepsy) and pheochromocytoma. Conversely, anxiety symptoms may be mistaken for features of physical disease, sometimes leading to unnecessary medical intervention.

Table I The features of anxiety

Psychologic	fear and apprehension
	inner tension and restlessness
	irritability
	impaired ability to concentrate
	increased startle response
	increased sensitivity to physical sensations
	disturbed sleep
Physical	increased muscle tension
	tremor
	sweating
	palpitations
	chest tightness and discomfort
	shortness of breath
	dry mouth
	difficulty swallowing
	diarrhea
	frequency of micturition
	loss of sexual interest
	dizziness
	numbness and tingling
	faintness

The ICD-10 and DSM-IV distinguish between the 'phobic' anxiety disorders, where anxiety is associated with particular situations, and other anxiety disorders, in which anxiety occurs in the absence of specific triggering events or circumstances. A distinction is also made between patients with and without panic attacks. The main anxiety disorders of DSM-IV are shown in Table 2.

GENERALIZED ANXIETY DISORDER

Generalized anxiety disorder (GAD) is characterized by unrealistic or excessive anxiety and worrying about a number of events or activities that are persistent (more than 6 months) and not restricted to particular circumstances (i.e. it is 'free-floating'). Common features include apprehension, with worries about future misfortune, inner tension and difficulty in concentrating; motor tension, with restlessness, tremor and headache; and autonomic anxiety, with excessive perspiration, dry mouth and epigastric discomfort. It is often associated with life events and environmental stress, and with physical illness. It may also be present in many patients with 'medically unexplained physical symptoms'. The DSM-IV criteria for the diagnosis of GAD are shown in Figure 5.3).

The prevalence of GAD in the general population aged between 15 and 54 years is approximately 5.1%. Twelve-month community prevalence rates are 2–4%. Primary care point prevalence is about 8%. The mean age of onset is approximately 35 years, and it is twice as common among women over 20 years[2,3].

The level of disability is similar to depression, and there is a strong association with physical illness. To differentiate the diagnosis from depressive illness, patients should be questioned about symptoms such as loss of interest and pleasure, loss of appetite and weight, diurnal variation in mood and early morning waking.

Table 2 The main anxiety disorders in DSM-IV

Panic disorder with or without agoraphobia
Agoraphobia without history of panic
Specific phobia
Social phobia
Obsessive–compulsive disorder (OCD)
Post-traumatic stress disorder (PTSD)
Acute stress disorder / acute situational anxiety
Generalized anxiety disorder (GAD)
Anxiety disorder due to a general medical disorder
Substance-induced anxiety disorder

PANIC DISORDER AND AGORAPHOBIA

Panic attacks

Panic attacks are discrete episodes of paroxysmal severe anxiety, and if they occur regularly in the absence of any obvious precipitating cause or other psychiatric diagnosis, panic disorder may be diagnosed. An early description of a panic attack was recorded by Sappho in the sixth century BC. Panic attacks are characterized by severe and frightening autonomic symptoms (e.g. shortness of breath, palpitations, excessive perspiration), dizziness, faintness and chest pain. Many seek a rapid escape (if possible) from the situation where the panic attack occurred. Panic attacks are usually of short duration (typically a few minutes), but many patients believe they are in imminent danger of death or collapse, and seek urgent medical attention.

Both panic attacks and agoraphobia are not 'codable' disorders within DSM-IV. In both cases the specific disorder in which they occur is coded (e.g. panic disorder without agoraphobia, panic disorder with agoraphobia and agoraphobia without history of panic disorder).

Panic disorder

Panic disorder can occur with or without agoraphobia. The prevalence of panic disorder varies (Figure 5.4), and it is characterized by the individual experiencing anxiety about being in places or situations from which escape might be difficult or embarrassing (see Figure 5.5). Typical fears include being outside the home, being in a crowd or standing in a queue, or using public transport. These feared situations are then avoided, or endured with marked distress, which is often lessened by the presence of a trusted companion. To be diagnosed as having panic disorder the individual must experience recurrent panic attacks that are not consistently associated with a specific situation or object and that often occur spontaneously. The panic attacks should not be associated with marked exertion or with exposure to dangerous or life-threatening situations.

A panic attack is characterized by a discrete episode of intense fear or discomfort, which starts abruptly, reaches a maximum intensity within a few minutes and lasts at least several minutes, with a minimum of four symptoms being present (including at least one autonomic symptom). The attack must not be caused by a physical disease, organic mental disorder, or other condition such as schizophrenia, mood disorder or somatoform disorder.

Comorbidity

Patients with panic attacks often present with somatic complaints or medically unexplained symptoms and there is a high use of medical services[4]. There is also some evidence that patients with panic disorder have an increased rate of mitral valve disease and thyroid disease. It is notable that men with panic disorder have an increased risk of cardiovascular mortality. There is a considerable overlap between panic disorder and depressive disorder, and most patients with panic disorder will experience a depressive episode at some point in their lives. In the World Health Organization collaborative study on psychological problems in general healthcare, 45.6% of patients with a history of panic attacks fulfilled ICD-10 diagnostic criteria for a current depressive episode or dysthymia[5]. Although the evidence is somewhat disputed, individuals with a lifetime diagnosis of panic disorder appear more likely to attempt suicide than subjects with no history of psychiatric disorder.

Agoraphobia

In the general population, agoraphobia can occur as an isolated condition, but in clinical samples it is invariably associated with panic disorder and often with coexisting major depression. The lifetime community prevalence of panic disorder, with or without agoraphobia, may be as high as 4.0%[6]. The point prevalence of panic disorder in primary care settings has been estimated as approximately 2.0%[6]. The lifetime prevalence rates of panic disorder are shown in Figure 5.4, while the diagnostic criteria for the diagnosis of panic disorder with agoraphobia are shown in Figure 5.6.

SPECIFIC (ISOLATED) PHOBIAS

The characteristic feature of a specific phobia (also known as isolated, or 'simple' phobia) is a single, discrete fear of a person (e.g. a dentist), a situation (e.g. flying) or an object (e.g. a particular animal). This fear causes significant emotional distress, and is often accompanied by marked avoidance. Although the lifetime prevalence of specific phobia in the general population may be as high as 11.3%, only a small proportion of sufferers seek medical treatment for their condition[1]. Most learn to live with the phobia, although occasionally treatment is sought when changes in lifestyle are necessary, such as when a promotion at work leads to the necessity for international travel.

SOCIAL PHOBIA

Social phobia (also known as social anxiety disorder) is characterized by an intense and persistent fear of being scrutinized or evaluated by other people (see Figure 5.7). The anxiety symptoms are restricted to, or predominate in, the feared situations or contemplation of the feared situations. The patient avoids such social situations, such as eating in public, writing in the presence of others, conversing with strangers and using public toilets due to a fear of being ridiculed or humiliated. Those with the disorder have a marked fear of being the focus of attention, or fear of behaving in a way that will be embarrassing or humiliating. In addition to more typical anxiety symptoms, at least one of the following must be present: blushing or shaking, fear of vomiting, urgency or fear of micturition or defecation.

There are two sub-types of social phobia:

- specific, when the feared situation is discrete (such as public speaking); and

- generalized, when it involves most social situations.

Social phobia usually begins in childhood or adolescence (about 90% before the age of 20) (see Figure 5.8). People with social phobia are less likely to marry and more likely to divorce than the general population. The prevalence is highest in people with a low socioeconomic status, probably reflecting the lower educational attainment and restricted career progression of affected individuals.

Until recently the condition was relatively unknown. The findings of the National Comorbidity Survey in the United States suggest that the 1-year prevalence among people aged 15–54 years is almost 8%, and the lifetime risk was calculated to be as high as 13.3%[1]. The disorder is more common in women than in men. There is a significant comorbidity with other disorders and also a significantly increased risk of suicide attempts. Patients with 'pure' social phobia are relatively uncommon in clinical settings.

Social phobia can be confused with panic disorder. In social phobia, panic attacks are restricted to feared social situations (or anticipation of those situations), whereas in panic disorder they occur unexpectedly in social encounters or when alone. In social phobia, patients fear appearing foolish and awkward, whereas in panic disorder patients fear losing control or death. In panic disorder, patients can enjoy social encounters when accompanied by a trusted friend; in social phobia, the presence of a friend or relative makes little difference. The avoidance of social situations can occur as a result of concerns about medical conditions, such as Parkinson's disease, benign essential tremor, stuttering, obesity and burns, but this should not be confused with social phobia.

POST-TRAUMATIC STRESS DISORDER

Post-traumatic stress disorder (PTSD) results from a person experiencing or witnessing a traumatic event (e.g. major accident, fire, sexual assault, physical assault and military combat). In the USA the lifetime prevalence is about 5% in men and 10% in women[7]. Women also suffer higher rates of sexual assault. A DSM-IV diagnosis requires a history of exposure to a 'traumatic event'. There are three main symptom clusters: intrusive recollections (thoughts, nightmares, flashbacks); avoidant behavior, numbing of emotions and hyper-arousal (increased anxiety and irritability, insomnia, poor concentration); and hypervigilence (see Figure 5.9). Nearly two-thirds of people with PTSD are 'chronic' sufferers. PTSD can present months or years after the traumatic event. It is also highly comorbid with other psychiatric problems, especially depression, anxiety and substance abuse or dependence.

OBSESSIVE–COMPULSIVE DISORDER

The characteristic features of obsessive–compulsive disorder (OCD) are obsessional thinking and compulsive behavior. Obsessive thinking includes recurrent persistent thoughts, impulses and images that cause marked anxiety or distress. Compulsive behavior include repetitive behavior, rituals or mental acts done to prevent or reduce anxiety. Other features include indecisiveness and inability to take action. Many patients with OCD experience significant degrees of anxiety, depression and

depersonalization (see Figure 5.10). OCD is uncommon in the general population, but minor obsessional symptoms are fairly common. The 1-month prevalence rates are estimated to be about 1% for men and 1.5% for women[8].

REFERENCES

1. Kessler RC, McGonagle KA, Zhao S, et al. Lifetime and 12-month prevalence of DSM-III-R psychiatric disorders in the United States: results from the National Comorbidity Survey. Arch Gen Psychiatry 1994;51:8–19

2. Kessler RC, DuPont RL, Berglund P, Wittchen HU. Impairment in pure and comorbid generalized anxiety disorder and major depression at 12 months in two national surveys. Am J Psychiatry 1999;156:1915–23

3. Wittchen HU, Carter RM, Pfister H, Montgomery SA, Kessler RC. Disabilities and quality of life in pure and comorbid generalized anxiety disorder and major depression in a national survey. Int Clin Psychopharmacol 2000;15:319–28

4. Katon W, Schulberg H. Epidemiology of depression in primary care. Gen Hosp Psychiatry 1992;14:237–47

5. Üstün TB, Sartorius. Mental Illness in General Health Care. Chichester, UK: John Wiley, 1995

6. Weissman MM, Bland RC, Canino GJ, et al. The cross-national epidemiology of panic disorder. Arch Gen Psychiatry 1997;54:305–9

7. Kessler RC, Sonnega A, Bromet E, Hughes M, Nelson CB. Posttraumatic stress disorder in the National Comorbidity Survey. Arch Gen Psychiatry 1995;52:1048–60

8. Bebbington PE. Epidemiology of obsessive-compulsive disorder. Br J Psychiatry 1998;35 (suppl):2–6

BIBLIOGRAPHY

Schneier FR, Johnson J, Hornig CD, Liebowitz MR, Weissman MM. Social phobia. Comorbidity and morbidity in an epidemiologic sample. Arch Gen Psychiatry 1992;49:282–8

CHAPTER 6

Suicide

INTRODUCTION

In the UK suicide is the sixth most frequent cause of death (after heart disease, cancer, respiratory disease, stroke and accidents), and is the third most common cause in the 15–44 year age group[1]. Suicide is the eighth most common cause of death in the US, while it is the second leading cause of death in the 25–34 age group (see Figure 6.1)[2]. Each year there are about 4000–5000 deaths by suicide in England and Wales, of which 400–500 involve overdoses of antidepressant drugs. Jick and colleagues[3] found 14% of overdoses in suicide (in the UK) resulted from the use of antidepressants. Figure 6.2 shows other studies that have assessed the rate of antidepressant overdose in suicide. A comparison of overdose deaths between antidepressant drugs is presented in Figure 6.3.

The rates of depression in an average general practitioner population of 2500 patients in shown in Figure 6.4. General practitioners have a role in the identification of suicide risk in those who have recently committed acts of deliberate self-harm. There are over 100 000 cases of deliberate self-harm in England and Wales per year. In the average practice with a population of 2500 there will be approximately three episodes of deliberate self-harm per year and one patient suicide every 5 years.

Factors associated with increased suicide risk after acts of deliberate self-harm (see Figure 6.5) include:

- act of deliberate self-harm planned long in advance;

- suicide note written;

- acts taken in anticipation of death (e.g. writing a will);

- being alone at the time of deliberate self-harm;

- patient making attempts to avoid discovery;

- not seeking help after deliberate self-harm;

- stating a wish to die;

- believing the act of deliberate self-harm would prove fatal;

- being sorry the act of deliberate self-harm failed; and

- continuing suicidal intent.

Two particular groups of patients are at significantly increased risk of suicide: those with a history of suicide attempts; and those recently discharged from psychiatric inpatient care. Community studies of suicide attempts are shown in Figure 6.6. About 1% of all deliberate self-harm patients commit suicide within 12 months of a suicide attempt, and up to 10% may eventually die by suicide[4]. In addition 10–15% of patients in contact with health services following a suicide attempt will eventually die by suicide, this risk being greatest during the first year after an attempt[4].

Up to 41% of suicide victims have received psychiatric inpatient care in the year prior to death, and up to 9% of suicide victims kill themselves within 1 day of discharge[5].

Those with depression have a greater risk of deliberate self-harm and suicide (see Figures 6.7 and 6.8). A recent meta-analysis estimated the standardized mortality ratio for completed suicide of those who had previously attempted suicide to be over 4000, higher than the risk attached to any particular psychiatric disorder, including major depression or alcoholism[6]. Other risk factors for suicide (see Figure 6.9) include:

- older age;

- male gender;

- single status;

- personality disorder;

- history of aggression;

- suicidal thoughts;

- social isolation;

- physical illness;

- alcohol abuse; and

- recent suicide attempt.

SUICIDE AND BEREAVEMENT

There is an increased risk of suicidal gestures, completed suicide and death from accidents following the death of a spouse or a parent[7–10]. The suicide risk for those widowed was first observed over a century ago by Durkheim who found that suicide was higher amongst those widowed compared to those married.

When compared to the general population Mergenhagen and colleagues[11] found the mortality ratio for suicide in young widowers (45–64 years of age) was about four and a half times the rate for married men of similar age. Most studies have found a gender bias with younger men being at the greatest risk of suicide[12], although Heikkinen and coworkers[13] found evidence of an association between widowhood and women aged 60–69 years.

A 12-year follow-up study in Washington, USA of 6266 white married and 3486 white widowed people aged 60 years and older found death rates from suicide to be 28.7 per 100 000 person years for the married and 40.4 for the widowed[14]. There was also a significant effect from gender with the suicide risk for widowed men estimated to be 3.3 times higher than that for married men, while the risk of suicide for widows and married women was found to be similar.

Several longitudinal studies have found that the risk of suicide is greatest for the period immediately following the loss. MacMahon and Pugh[9] compared 320 widowed people who had committed suicide to a matched sample of widows who had died from non-suicide causes. They found that, although the risk of suicide among the widowed population was generally higher in the first 4 years after the death of the spouse, the risk of suicide in the first year was 2.5 times higher, and in the first, second and third years about 1.5 times higher. The risk at 4

years or more was equal to that of the control group. The age-standardized suicide rate was 3.5 times higher for widowed men than married men. Widows had twice the risk compared to those who were married.

Based on MacMahon and Pugh's findings, Duberstein and colleagues[15] used the psychologic autopsy method as a way of distinguishing those who committed suicide more than 4 years after the death of their spouse compared to those who committed suicide within 4 years. Although using small numbers ($n = 21$, > 4 years; $n = 14$, < 4 years), they found those who committed suicide within 4 years had significantly higher rates of psychiatric treatment, earlier loss or separation from one or both parents and a non-significant ($P = 0.07$) higher rate of substance abuse. Interestingly, loss of a close interpersonal relationship (including bereavement and separation) is a significant predictor of suicide in alcoholics[16].

REFERENCES

1. McClure GM. Changes in suicide in England and Wales, 1960-1997. Br J Psychiatry 2000;176:64–7

2. Centers for Disease Control and Prevention. Leading Causes of Death Reports. Washington, DC: CDC, 2000: http://webapp.cdc.gov/sasweb/ncipc/leadcaus.html

3. Jick SS, Dean AD, Jick H. Antidepressants and suicide. Br Med J 1995;310:215–18

4. Cullberg J, Wasserman D, Stefansson CG. Who commits suicide after a suicide attempt? Acta Psychiatrica Scand 1988;77:598-603.

5. Pirkis J, Burgess P. Suicide and recency of health care contacts. A systematic review. Br J Psychiatry 1998;173:462–74

6. Harris EC, Barraclough B. Suicide as an outcome for mental disorders. Br J Psychiatry 1997;170:205–28

7. Kaprio J, Koskenvuo M, Rita H. Mortality after bereavement: a prospective study of 95,647 widowed persons. Am J Public Health 1987;77:283–7

8. Bunch J. Recent bereavement in relation to suicide. J Psychosom Res 1972;16:361–6

9. Bunch J, Barraclough B. The influence of parental death anniversairies upon suicide dates. Br J Psychiatry 1971; 118:621

10. MacMahon B, Pugh TF. Suicide in the widowed. Am J Epidemiol 1965;81:23–31

11. Mergenhagen PM, Lee BA, Gove WR. Till death do us part: recent changes in the relationship between marital status and mortality. Sociol Social Res 1985;70:53–6

12. Gove WR. Sex, marital status, and suicide. J Health Social Behavior 1972;13:204–13

13. Heikkinen ME, Isometsa ET, Marttunen MJ, Aro HM,

Lonnqvist JK. Social factors in suicide. *Br J Psychiatry* 1995;167:747–53

14. Li G. The interaction effect of bereavement and sex on the risk of suicide in the elderly: an historical cohort study. *Soc Sci Med* 1995;40:825–8

15. Duberstein PR, Conwell Y, Cox C. Suicide in widowed persons. *Am J Geriatr Psychiatry* 1998;6:328–34

16. Murphy GE, *et al.* Suicide and alcoholism: Interpersonal loss confirmed as a predictor. *Arch Gen Psychiatry* 1979;36:65–9

BIBLIOGRAPHY

Angst J. Hypomania. Apropos of a cohort of young patients [in French]. *Encephale* 1992;18:23–9

Arato M, Demeter E, Rihmer Z, Somogyi E. Retrospective psychiatric assessment of 200 suicides in Budapest. *Acta Psychiatr Scand* 1988;77:454–6

Asgard U. A psychiatric study of suicide among urban Swedish women. *Acta Psychiatr Scand* 1990;82:115–24

Barraclough B, Bunch J, Nelson B, Sainsbury P. A hundred cases of suicide: clinical aspects. *Br J Psychiatry* 1974;125:355–73

Brent DA, Perper JA, Moritz G, *et al.* Psychiatric risk factors for adolescent suicide: a case-control study. *J Am Acad Child Adolesc Psychiatry* 1993;32:521–9

Breslau N, Davis GC, Andreski P. Migraine, psychiatric disorders, and suicide attempts: an epidemiologic study of young adults. *Psychiatry Res* 1991;37:11–23

Dorpat TL, Ripley HS. A study of suicide in the Seattle area. *Comp Psychiatry* 1960;1:349–59

Dyck RJ, Bland RC, Newman SC, Orn H. Suicide attempts and psychiatric disorders in Edmonton. *Acta Psychiatr Scand* 1988;338 (suppl):64–71

Harris EC, Barraclough B. Suicide as an outcome for mental disorders. A meta-analysis. *Br J Psychiatry* 1997;170:205–28

Henriksson MM, Aro HM, Marttunen MJ, *et al.* Mental disorders and comorbidity in suicide. *Am J Psychiatry* 1993;150:935–40

Henry JA, Alexander CA, Sener EK. Relative mortality from overdose of antidepressants. *Br Med J* 1995;310:221–4

Isacsson G, Bergman U, Rich CL. Antidepressants, depression and suicide: an analysis of the San Diego study. *J Affect Disord* 1994;32:277–86

Isacsson G, Holmgren P, Wasserman D, Bergman U. Use of antidepressants among people committing suicide in Sweden. *Br Med J* 1994;308:506–9

Isacsson G, Holmgren P, Druid H, Bergman U. The utilization of antidepressants – a key issue in the prevention of suicide: an analysis of 5281 suicides in Sweden during the period 1992–1994. *Acta Psychiatr Scand* 1997;96:94–100

Isometsa ET, Henriksson MM, Aro HM, Heikkinen ME, Kuoppasalmi KI, Lonnqvist JK. Suicide in major depression. *Am J Psychiatry* 1994;151:530–6

Levy JC, Deykin EY. Suicidality, depression, and substance abuse in adolescence. *Am J Psychiatry* 1989;146:1462–7

Manz R, Valentin E, Schepank H. Social support and psychogenic disease. Results of an epidemiologic field study [in German]. *Z Psychosom Med Psychoanal* 1987;33:162–70

Marttunen MJ, Aro HM, Henriksson MM, Lonnqvist JK. Mental disorders in adolescent suicide. DSM-III-R axes I and II diagnoses in suicides among 13- to 19-year-olds in Finland. *Arch Gen Psychiatry* 1991;48:834–9

Moscicki EK, O'Carroll P, Rae DS, Locke BZ, Roy A, Regier DA. Suicide attempts in the Epidemiologic Catchment Area Study. *Yale J Biol Med* 1988;61:259–68

Paykel ES, Myers JK, Lindenthal JJ, Tanner J. Suicidal feelings in the general population: a prevalence study. *Br J Psychiatry* 1974;124:460–9

Ramsay R, Bagley C. The prevalence of suicidal behaviors, attitudes and associated social experiences in an urban population. *Suicide Life Threat Behav* 1985;15:151–67

Rich CL, Young D, Fowler RC. San Diego suicide study. I. Young vs old subjects. *Arch Gen Psychiatry* 1986;43:577–82

Rich CL, Isacsson G. Suicide and antidepressants in south Alabama: evidence for improved treatment of depression. *J Affect Disord* 1997;45:135–42

Schepank H. Epidemiology of psychogenic disorders. Results of a field study in the Federal Republic of Germany. Berlin: Springer Verlag, 1987

Schwab JJ, Warheit GJ, Holzer CE III. Suicidal ideation and behavior in a general population. *Dis Nerv Syst* 1972;33:745–8

Velez CN, Cohen P. Suicidal behavior and ideation in a community sample of children: maternal and youth reports. *J Am Acad Child Adolesc Psychiatry* 1988;27:349–56

Wacker HR. Reported in Angst J, Degonda M, Ernst C. The Zurich Study: XV. Suicide attempts in a cohort from age 20 to 30. *Eur Arch Psychiatry Clin Neurosci* 1992;242:135–41

CHAPTER 7

Causes of depression

INTRODUCTION

Depression has many causes (see Figures 7.1 and 7.2), which include:

- genetic factors;

- neurotransmitter disturbances; and

- psychosocial factors:

    adverse experiences in childhood;

    chronic major difficulties;

    undesirable life events;

    limited social network; and

    low self-esteem.

In most patients, depressive episodes arise from the combination of familial, biological, psychologic and social factors, operating over time and progressively increasing the risk of developing a depressive disorder. Depressed mood also occurs in certain physical illnesses (see Figure 7.3) and as a part of many different psychiatric syndromes, e.g. anxiety disorders, alcohol abuse, substance abuse and eating disorders (see Tables 1 and 2 and Figure 7.4).

GENETIC FACTORS

Genetic influences are most marked in patients with more severe forms of depressive disorder and 'biological' symptoms. The morbid risk in first-degree relatives is increased in all studies, this elevation being independent of the effects of environment or upbringing (see Figure 7.5). In less severe forms of depression, genetic factors are less significant and environmental factors relatively more important.

Potential genetic markers for affective disorders have been localized to chromosomes X, 4, 5, 11, 18 and 21. Some of these sites have been linked to the neurobiology of depression: for example, two of the putative markers on the long arm of chromosome 5 contain candidate genes contributing to the receptors for norepinephrine, dopamine, γ-amino butyric acid and glutamate[1].

The genetic 'loading' for bipolar illness seems greater than that for unipolar depression. First-degree relatives of patients with bipolar disorder have a 5–10 times greater risk of developing a mood disorder, compared

Table 1 Examples of physical illness associated with depression

malignancy
hepatitis
glandular fever and other chronic infections
Parkinson's disease
multiple sclerosis
dementia
endocrine disease (thyroid disorders, Addison's disease)
hypercalcemia
rheumatoid arthritis
systemic lupus erythematosus (SLE)
cancer
acquired immune deficiency syndrome (AIDS)
cardio- and cerebrovascular disease

Table 2 Drugs that can cause symptoms of depression

β-blockers
anticonvulsants
calcium channel blockers
corticosteroids
oral contraceptives
antipsychotic drugs
drugs used for Parkinson's disease (e.g. levodopa)
alcohol

with unrelated individuals[2]. The concordance rate for bipolar disorder among monozygotic (identical) twins is approximately 70%. However, attempts to identify definite genetic markers for the condition have not been successful[3]. Approximately 25% of cases of bipolar illness in families with multiple cases may be linked to a locus near the centromere on chromosome 18, and as much as 20% to a locus on chromosome 21q22.3[4]. However, there is no single cause for bipolar affective disorder and, like unipolar depression, individual episodes usually result from the combination of familial, biological, psychologic and social factors.

NEUROTRANSMITTER DISTURBANCES

There is evidence that abnormalities in the level or function of the serotonin (5-hydroxytryptamine, 5-HT), norepinephrine and dopamine neurotransmitters acting on central nervous system neurons may be important in the pathophysiology of depression, although this evidence is inconclusive. Animal studies indicate that serotonin is intimately involved in the regulation of the sleep–wake cycle, appetite, sexual behavior and aggression. Patients with major depression appear to have abnormal serotonergic neurotransmission (see Figures 7.6–7.8). Some of these abnormalities (such as increased numbers of platelet and brain 5-HT$_2$-receptors) appear to be linked to suicidal or impulsive behavior, rather than to the depressive syndrome *per se*. The results of neuroendocrine studies suggest that depression is associated with decreased neurotransmission at postsynaptic 5-HT$_{1A}$ receptors (see Figures 7.9 and 7.10). Many antidepressants are thought to produce their therapeutic effects by acting upon these postsynaptic 5-HT$_{1A}$ receptors.

Depression is also associated with increased 24-h adrenocorticotropic hormone (ACTH) levels, as well as elevated urinary and plasma cortisol levels. Exogenous administration of ACTH leads to a greater release of cortisol whilst the patient is depressed, suggesting a state-dependent oversensitive adrenal gland (Figure 7.11). Recent research indicates that depression is associated with enlargement of the adrenal glands, which shrink in size following adequate treatment. Some of the changes in brain 5-HT function seen in depressed patients may themselves result from hypersecretion of cortisol[5].

Abnormalities of noradrenergic and dopaminergic neurotransmission are also important in the etiology of depression. Animal studies suggest norepinephrine plays a major role in maintaining arousal and drive. Although there is no consistent change in noradrenergic receptor function in patients with depression, down-regulation of α$_2$ somatodendritic receptors by antidepressant drugs may underlie the treatment response (Figures 7.12 and 7.13)[6]. Dopaminergic dysfunction has been reported in psychotic and bipolar depression, seasonal affective disorder and depression associated with Parkinson's disease. Antidepressants may resolve anhedonia and loss of drive by increasing the sensitization of dopamine D$_2$ and D$_3$ receptors. Manic episodes may be associated with overactivity in dopamine pathways within the brain, as mania can be provoked by dopamine-releasing psychostimulants, such as cocaine and amphetamine. Depressed bipolar patients may be more likely to respond than unipolar patients to dopamine-enhancing agents. such as bromocriptine or levodopa. Manic episodes occurring after childbirth have been linked to abnormalities in the release of growth hormone that follows challenge with dopamine-releasing investigational compounds[7].

Structural and functional abnormalities of the brain

There have been no adequate controlled post-mortem studies of brain structure in bipolar illness. *In vivo* studies using magnetic resonance imaging and computerized assisted tomography suggest that the brains of some bipolar patients may have enlarged lateral and third ventricles, and an increase in the ventricle–brain ratio (see Figures 7.14–7.16). However, these abnormalities are not reported consistently[8], and are less marked than those seen in many patients with schizophrenia. Studies of brain function, using positron-emission tomography or single-photon emission computed tomography have also produced variable results, but no brain area has been shown to have consistently reduced or increased function (see Figures 7.17–7.20), although there is some evidence that points to reduced bilateral perfusion to the frontotemporal cortex.

Repeated episodes of affective illness in bipolar disorder may lead to long-term changes in neuronal systems involved in the regulation of mood. This in turn may reduce the threshold for further episodes of illness. This 'kindling' model has been used to explain the sensitization seen in some patients with epilepsy, and is now being applied to bipolar illness. The first episodes of illness may be related to stressful life events, but successive episodes lead to biochemical changes that render the patient ever more susceptible to other life stresses. The process of sensitization continues until affective episodes arise spontaneously. This may explain the increase in frequency of episodes with time, seen in many bipolar patients[9,10] and could also explain why anticonvulsant drugs are often effective[11].

PSYCHOSOCIAL FACTORS

Low self-esteem, an obsessional personality, the experience of adversity in childhood and maladaptive negative patterns of thinking about oneself and others, are all recognized psychologic 'risk factors' for depression. Other factors include excessive undesirable recent life events, usually involving loss (such as bereavement, divorce and redundancy), and persisting major difficulties, including being a lone parent, overcrowding, prolonged unemployment, poverty and lack of social support or intimacy.

Psychosocial factors, particularly family dynamics, are undoubtedly important in influencing the course of bipolar illness once established. However, their role in causing the condition to appear is unclear.

It seems probable that 'vulnerability' factors, such as the lack of an intimate confiding relationship or caring for three or more children under the age of 15 years at home, confer a predisposition to depression when coupled with threatening life events or chronic social stress.

REFERENCES

1. Souery D, Lipp O, Matieu B, Mendlewicz J. Advances in the genetics of depression. In: Honig A, van Praag HM, eds. *Depression: Neurobiological, Psychopathological and Therapeutic Advances*. Chichester, UK: John Wiley, 1997:297–309

2. Craddock N, Jones I. Genetics of bipolar disorder. *J Med Genet* 1999;36:585–94

3. Holmes C, Lovestone S. The molecular genetics of mood disorders. *Curr Opin Psychiatry* 1997;10:79–83

4. Berretini W. Genetic studies of bipolar disorders: new and recurrent findings. *Molec Psychiatry* 1996;1:172–3

5. Cowen PJ, Smith KA. Serotonin and depression. In: Honig A, van Praag HM, eds. *Depression: Neurobiological, Psychopathological and Therapeutic Advances*. Chichester, UK: John Wiley, 1997:129–46

6. Anand A, Charney DS. Catecholamines in depression. In: Honig A, van Praag HM, eds. *Depression: Neurobiological, Psychopathological and Therapeutic Advances*. Chichester, UK: John Wiley, 1997:147–78

7. Wieck A, Kumar R, Hirst AD, Marks MN, Campbell IC, Checkley SA. Increased sensitivity of dopamine receptors and recurrence of affective illness after childbirth. *Br Med J* 1991;303:613–16

8. Norris SDK, Krishnan RR, Ahearn E. Structural changes in the brain of patients with bipolar affective disorder by MRI: a review of the literature. *Prog Neuropsychopharmacol Biol Psychiatry* 1997;21:1323–37

9. Angst J. Course of affective disorders. In: Van Praag HM, Lader HM, Rafaelson OJ, Sachar EJ, eds. *Handbook of Biological Psychiatry*. New York: Marcel Dekker, 1981:225–42

10. Zis AP, Grof P, Webster M, *et al.* The cyclicity of affective disorders and its modification by drugs. *Psychopharmacology (Berl)* 1980;16:47–9

11. Post RM, Rubinow DR, Ballenger JC. Conditioning and sensitisation in the longitudinal course of affective illness. *Br J Psychiatry* 1986;149:191–201

CHAPTER 8

The need for long-term treatment of depression

INTRODUCTION

Both unipolar depression and bipolar affective disorder should be regarded as potentially lifelong episodic conditions. The focus of treatment should be as much on long-term management as on short-term relief of symptoms. The efficacy of most new antidepressants and some psychologic therapies, in continuation and maintenance treatment, has been evaluated, and most treatments have been found beneficial. However, long-term benefit cannot be assumed: for example, there is currently no good evidence to support the use of either nortriptyline or mianserin in prolonged treatment.

A model that is commonly employed when treating patients with major depression in secondary care has been proposed[1]. Initial acute treatment results in a significant reduction of depressive symptoms (response), followed by progression to the premorbid state, with absence of symptoms (remission). Stable remission for 4–6 months is thought to constitute a recovery from depression. A worsening of symptoms or return of major depression is called relapse if it occurs before recovery has been achieved, and recurrence if it occurs later. Relapses are assumed to represent inadequate treatment of the index depressive episode, whereas recurrence represents a new episode of illness.

Treatment therefore consists of three phases (Figure 8.1). Acute treatment lasts until remission, continuation treatment from remission to recovery and maintenance (or prophylaxis) from recovery onwards. This model has merits in secondary care, but its application to the long-term treatment of depressive symptoms in primary care is not yet proven.

LENGTH OF CONTINUATION TREATMENT

Evidence from predominantly secondary care settings indicates that over one-third of patients with major depression experience a relapse of depression in the first year after remission of symptoms. Most relapses occur in the first 4 months in younger adults, but in elderly patients the risk of relapse extends more steadily over 12 months[2]. The risk of relapse in primary care is not established, although a relapse rate of 37% has been described[3]. A meta-analysis of controlled studies in which patients with major depression were treated for 2–6 months beyond the point of remission has shown that antidepressants halve the risk of relapse[4]. Typically 50% of patients receiving placebo relapse, compared with 20–25% on antidepressant drugs. Most relapses occur in the first 3–4 months of treatment (see Figures 8.2 and 8.3)[5]. For these reasons, it has been recommended that antidepressant drugs should be continued for at least 6 months after remission of major depression (see Figures 8.4 and 8.5)[6].

LENGTH OF MAINTENANCE TREATMENT

There is some uncertainty about the duration of maintenance or prophylactic treatment in recurrent unipolar depression. Controlled studies in predominantly secondary care patients with recurrent depressive episodes have shown that maintenance treatment after recovery reduces the risk of recurrence over the next 1–5 years[7]. For example, in a study that examined the efficacy of 3 years' maintenance treatment with the tricyclic antidepressant imipramine, relapse rates were 80% in those switched to placebo, compared to 20% in those remaining on imipramine[8]. It has been recommended that maintenance treatment should continue for at least 5 years in patients who have experienced three or more episodes of major depression in 5 years, or more than a total of five episodes[6]. The situation is less clear for bipolar depression, where lengthening the duration of antidepressant treatment can sometimes precipitate hypomanic or manic episodes, or contribute to 'cycle acceleration', in which episodes of illness become more frequent over time.

REFERENCES

1. Frank E, Prien RF, Jarret RB, et al. Conceptualization and rationale for consensus definitions of terms in major depressive disorder. Remission, recovery, relapse and recurrence. Arch Gen Psychiatry 1991;48:851–5

2. Belsher G, Costello CG. Relapse after recovery from unipolar depression: a critical review. Psychol Bull 1988;194:84–96

3. Lin EHB, Katon WJ, Von Korff M, et al. Relapse of depression in primary care: rate and clinical predictors. Arch Fam Med 1998;7:443–9

4. Loonen AJ, Peer PG, Zwanikken GJ. Continuation and maintenance therapy with antidepressive agents. Meta-analysis of research. Pharm Week Sci 1991;13:167–75

5. Reimherr FW, Amsterdam HD, Quitkin FM, et al. Optimal length of continuation therapy in depression: a prospective assessment during long-term treatment with fluoxetine. Am J Psychiatry 1998;155:1247–53

6. Anderson IM, Nutt DJ, Deakin JFW. Evidence-based guidelines for treating depressive illness with antidepressants: a revision of the 1993 British Association for Psychopharmacology guidelines. J Psychopharmacol 2000;14:3–20

7. Montgomery SA. Long-term treatment of depression. Br J Psychiatry 1994;165 (suppl 26):31–6

8. Frank E, Kupfer DJ, Perel JM, Cornes C, Jarrett DB, Mallinger AG, Thase ME, McEachran AB, Grochocinski VJ. Three-year outcomes for maintenance therapies in recurrent depression. Arch Gen Psychiatry 1990;47:1093–9

BIBLIOGRAPHY

Dunn RL, Donoghue JM, Ozminkowski RJ, Stephenson D, Hylan TR. Longitudinal patterns of antidepressant prescribing in primary care in the UK: comparison with treatment guidelines. J Psychopharmacol 1999;13:136–43

Russell JM, Berndt ER, Miceli R, Colucci S, Grudzinski AN. Course and cost of treatment for depression with fluoxetine, paroxetine, and sertraline. Am J Manag Care 1999;5:597–606

CHAPTER 9

Antidepressant drugs

INTRODUCTION

Recent evidence-based guidelines from the British Association for Psychopharmacology[1] state that doctors should "match choice of antidepressant drug to individual patient requirements as far as possible, taking into account likely short-term and long-term effects" and further "in the absence of special factors, choose antidepressants which are better tolerated, safer in overdose and more likely to be prescribed at effective doses."

The antidepressant drugs that are available currently include the tricyclic antidepressants (TCAs), monoamine oxidase inhibitors (MAOIs), reversible inhibitors of monoamine oxidase type A (RIMAs) selective serotonin re-uptake inhibitors (SSRIs), serotonin and norepinephrine re-uptake inhibitors (SNRIs), norepinephrine and serotonin selective antidepressants (NESSA), norepinephrine re-uptake inhibitors (NERI) and several other compounds. However, the antidepressant drugs are not ideal and each drug has its own side-effect profile, which limits its use in some patients (see Table 1).

THE IDEAL ANTIDEPRESSANT

The ideal antidepressant would fulfil a range of criteria (Figure 9.1), including that they should:

- be effective across a range of depressive disorders;

- be effective in short-term and long-term treatments;

- be effective across a range of age groups;

- have a rapid onset of action;

- involve once-daily dosage;

- be cost-effective;

- be well tolerated;

- have no behavioral toxicity;

- be suitable in the physically ill;

- be free from interactions with food or drugs; and

- be safe in overdose.

When starting treatment with antidepressant drugs, it can be helpful to follow a fairly simple protocol, designed to offer the best chance of choosing the right treatment, and using it effectively and sensitively. Clearly, no two patients have identical problems, and clinical judgement is always required when making treatment decisions for individual patients.

STARTING TREATMENT WITH ANTIDEPRESSANTS

When a patient has been identified as benefiting from drug treatment, the following criteria should be observed:

- establish the presence of a depressive disorder;

- exclude another underlying severe mental disorder (e.g. schizophrenia);

- determine the severity of depression:

    psychosis (refer to psychiatric services);

    severe (refer to psychiatric services);

    moderate (start on antidepressants); or

    mild (review the patient later).

- establish whether physical illness is present;

- choose an effective, well-tolerated, safe antidepressant;

- warn the patient about possible side-effects;

Table 1 The adverse effects and problematic interactions of antidepressants

Class of antidepressant drugs	Examples	Adverse effects	Problematic interactions
Tricyclic antidepressants	Amitryptiline Amoxepine Clomipramine Dothiepin Doxepin Imipramine Lofepramine Nortriptyline	*Anticholinergic:* dry mouth, constipation, urinary retention, accomodation problems, glaucoma *Antihistaminergic:* sedation *Alpha blockade:* postural hypotension, sedation *Unknown mechanism:* weight gain *Cardiotoxic:* QT prolongation, ST elevation, AV block, membrane stabilization, arrythmias Neurotoxic: delirium, movement disorders, convulsions	MAOIs (esp. clomipramine and tranylcypromine) Antiepileptics, barbiturates decrease TCA levels Cimetidine increases TCA levels Warfarin action potentiated Alcohol potentiates TCA sedation
Related compounds to tricyclic anti-depressants	Maprotiline Mianserin	Cardiotoxic, may precipitate seizures in those patients predisposed to epilepsy. Low cardiotoxicity, drowsiness, dizziness, weight gain, dyspepsia and nausea. Lowering of white cell count and fatal agranulocytosis has been reported. Rare side-effects of mianserin include arthritis and hepatitis	Similar to TCA above Drowsiness enhanced by alcohol
Monoamine oxidase inhibitors (MAOIs)	Phenelzine Isocarboxazid Tranylcypromine	Hypertensive crisis occurs with tyramine-containing foods and some drugs. Tyramine normally inactivated in the gut by MAO acts by releasing NE Symptoms - flushing, headache, increased BP, rarely CVA Foods – e.g. cheese, yoghurt, yeast extracts, meat, alcohol, broad beans, pickled herrings	Tyramine Sympathomimetics (include cold remedies) Other antidepressants Pethidine Alcohol, barbiturates, ?anesthetics: CNS depression Insulin: impared blood glucose control
Reversible inhibitors of monoamine oxidase type A isoenzyme (RIMA)	Moclobemide	Tyramine pressor response (lower risk than MAOIs) Agitation, anxiety and excitability, dizziness, nausea and sleep disturbances	Potentiates ephedrine and the serotonergic effects of pethidine. Cimetidine decreases the hepatic metabolism of moclobemide. In theory, combining SSRIs with moclobemide can produce the 'serotonin syndrome' (including agitation, confusion, myoclonus, hyperthermia and incoordination. Caution when combined with the TCA clomipramine or the SSRI citalopram Useful interactions (with caution): TCA's lithium
Selective serotonin re-uptake inhibitors SSRIs	Fluoxetine Paroxetine Sertraline Citalopram Fluvoxamine	Nausea/vomiting – early (FLUV) Agitation – early (FLUO) Akathisia – early Parkinsonism – uncommon Sedation/dizziness – 10-20% Convulsions – rare Sexual dysfunction – common (M&F) Discontinuation symptoms	MAOIs L-tryptophan With fluvoxamine (due to CYP1A2 inhibition) caffeine, clozapine, theophylline With fluoxetine and paroxetine (due to CYP2D6 inhibition) beta blockers, neuroleptics, opiates, TCAs

continued over

Table 1 continued The adverse effects and problematic interactions of antidepressants

Class of antidepressant drugs	Examples	Adverse effects	Problematic interactions
Serotonin and norepinephrine re-uptake inhibitor (SNRI)	Venlafaxine	Nausea, dizziness, sleep disturbances, dry mouth, headache, nervousness. Overdose may result in cardiovascular toxicity, central nervous system depression and seizures. Rise in blood pressure and possible hypertension. Discontinuation effects: mainly headache, nausea and dizziness	Co-administration of cimetidine inhibits the first-pass metabolism of venlafaxine. Risk of serotonin syndrome with MAOIs. Modest inhibitory effects on the cytochrome P450 system enzymes
Norepinephrine and serotonin-selective antidepressant (NESSA)	Mirtazapine	Sedation, increased appetite, weight gain	Enhanced sedation with alcohol and benzodiazepines
Phenylpiperazines	Trazodone	Excessive sedation, nausea, postural hypotension, priapism (about 1 in 6000 men)	Enhanced sedation with alcohol. Thioridazine may increase trazodone levels
	Nefazodone	Nausea, restlessness	Risk of fatal ventricular arrythmias via inhibition of CYP3A4 when combined with astemizole, terfenadine or cisapride
Norepinephrine re-uptake inhibitor (NERI)	Reboxetine	Dry mouth, constipation, increased sweating, urinary hesitancy (mainly men). Should not be prescribed to men with prostatic enlargement. Transient increase in blood pressure: caution in patients with cardiac disease, and in those taking antihypertensives	Should be used cautiously with drugs that are metabolized by CYP3A4 (e.g. antiarrhythmic drugs), and avoided with drugs that potently inhibit CYP3A4
Thioxanthene	Tryptophan	Eosinophilia–myalgia syndrome (EMS), sedation and myoclonus	Serotonin syndrome when combined with SSRIs

- prescribe at low dose for 1–2 days, then increase to an effective dose;
- review adherence and side-effects within 1 week; and
- evaluate efficacy at around 4 weeks.

Figure 9.2 summarizes the criteria for starting patients on antidepressants.

TRICYCLIC ANTIDEPRESSANTS

Most TCAs can cause drowsiness and interfere with work, and can be dangerous when taken in overdose (see Figure 9.3). It has been argued by some that TCA presciptions should be initiated only by psychiatrists (see Table 1).

TCA efficacy

TCAs are used in the acute treatment of episodes of depression. They produce a 55–70% response rate with a 10–20 day delay[1]. They are useful in relapse prevention and are effective, but need an adequate dose and there may be problems with compliance. TCAs are especially useful in patients who are agitated, retarded or have severe illness, but are less useful in elderly patients, patients with psychotic depression or the physically ill.

TCAs should be avoided in younger patients, elderly patients, patients who drive, when drowsiness is unacceptable, when there is a risk of suicide attempts, when the therapeutic dose is not feasible, when there is pre-existing cardiac disease or when long-term treatment is needed.

TCAs are useful in cases where there has been a previous response to TCA treatment and when that previous treatment was well accepted. TCAs are also useful when there is no risk of suicide attempts, when drowsiness is acceptable or preferable and when the patient is able to tolerate a recommended dose (see Figures 9.4 and 9.5).

Pharmacology of TCAs

TCA pharmacology involves a number of interconnected effects on the nervous system (see Figure 9.6):

- 5-HT re-uptake inhibition and 5-HT receptor effects;

- norepinephrine (NE) re-uptake inhibition;

- anticholinergic effects;

- antihistaminergic effects; and

- adrenergi c effects.

TCA pharmacokinetics

TCAs are rapidly absorbed and widely distributed, while there is genetic variation in liver metabolism. Tertiary amines are generally more potent at blocking 5-HT uptake, while secondary amines are more potent at blocking NE uptake. Tertiary amines are metabolized to secondary amines (e.g. amitriptyline to nortriptyline and imipramine to desmethylimipramine). Discontinuation effects (cholinergic hyperfunction) can occur with TCAs.

Figure 9.7 describes the side-effects typically seen with TCAs.

MONOAMINE OXIDASE INHIBITORS

Examples of monoamine oxidase inhibitors (MAOIs) include phenelzine, isocarboxazid and tranylcypromine (Figure 9.8).

Stringent dietary restrictions are necessary in patients taking traditional MAOIs, as naturally occurring monoamines (such as tyramine in cheese) and sympathomimetics in cough and cold medicines can interact with MAOIs to produce a fatally catastrophic hypertension.

MAOI efficacy

MAOIs are often used in cases of severe depression, especially those associated with lethargy and poor motivation. They are also used in cases where treatment resistance is seen (possibly also combined with lithium and/or L-tryptophan). Anxiety states can be treated with

MAOIs, and they are sometimes helpful in borderline personality disorder.

In association with mood stabilizers, MAOIs are given to those with bipolar disorder. They are also prescribed in certain cases of atypical depression. Dosage needs to be adequate (e.g. phenelzine 75–90 mg/day)

MAOI neurochemistry

Figure 9.9 shows the known actions of MAOIs on the nervous system, which can be summarized as follows:

- irreversible inhibition of MAO-A (and -B);

- MAO-A metabolizes NE, 5-HT and tyramine;

- MAO-B metabolizes DA, tyramine and phenylethylamine;

- increases stores and release of 5-HT and NE; and

- sympathomimetic effects (e.g. tranylcypromine).

Reported side-effects are shown in Figure 9.10.

MAOI pharmacokinetics

MAOIs are characterized by rapid absorption, but toxic levels can occur in the slow acetylators. The half-life is not as important as the time taken to replace stores of MAO after irreversible blockade.

REVERSIBLE INHIBITORS OF MONOAMINE OXIDASE TYPE A

Moclobemide

Moclobemide is a RIMA, with proven efficacy and acceptable tolerability in the short-term treatment of depression (see Figures 9.11 and 9.12)[2]. It was the first RIMA to enter widespread clinical use. In development, it was expected that selective inhibition of MAO-A by moclobemide would avoid the stringent dietary requirements of nonselective MAOIs. In principle, the MAO-B should be free to metabolize tyramine contained within food and the reversibility of RIMAs should allow tyramine to displace it from MAO-A binding sites.

A review of randomized controlled trials show that, at daily doses of 300–600 mg, moclobemide has comparable efficacy to the TCAs imipramine, clomipramine and amitriptyline, and to the SSRIs fluoxetine and fluvoxamine[3]. Subgroup analysis of the clinical trial database indicates that moclobemide is efficacious in the short-term treatment of unipolar, bipolar, 'endogenous' and 'reactive' depression[4]. In some countries moclobemide has a license for the treatment of social phobia (social anxiety disorder)[5,6], although only two out of four randomized controlled trials found it to be significantly more effective than placebo[7].

Studies in healthy volunteers have shown that short-term treatment with high doses of moclobemide (900–1200 mg/day) can produce an exaggerated tyramine pressor response, and that a standard dose (300 mg twice-daily) can potentiate the effects of ephedrine on heart rate and blood pressure[8,9]. For these reasons, there should be caution when coprescribing potentially interacting medications. Patients should be advised to avoid consuming large amounts of tyramine-rich foodstuffs. Moclobemide has a low incidence of sexual dysfunction.

SELECTIVE SEROTONIN REUPTAKE INHIBITORS

Examples of the SSRIs in common use are fluoxetine, fluvoxamine, paroxetine, sertraline, citalopram and escitalopram (Figure 9.13).

Compared to TCAs and MAOIs, SSRIs are somewhat better tolerated and relatively safer, but treatment-emergent insomnia and sexual dysfunction are common problems. In United Kingdom primary care, the most commonly prescribed antidepressants are the TCAs (including the older drugs amitriptyline and dothiepin, and the newer TCA lofepramine) and SSRIs. Systematic reviews and meta-analyses suggest that the different classes of antidepressant drugs have comparable overall efficacy[1,10–12]. SSRIs appear marginally less effective than TCAs in hospitalized patients with major depression, but they have similar efficacy to tricyclic drugs in the majority of patients, seen in primary care or outpatient settings[1,10–12].

Advantages and disadvantages of SSRIs

SSRIs have a number of advantages in the treatment of depression and the associated disorders:

- broad-spectrum efficacy (depression, panic disorder, obsessive–compulsive disorder (OCD), social anxiety disorder and post-traumatic stress disorder);

- reduced adverse-event burden;

- safety in overdose; and

- prescribed in therapeutic doses.

Nevertheless, SSRIs are not necessarily without their disadvantages:

- reduced efficacy in depressed inpatients;

- some common adverse events (gastrointestinal upset, sexual dysfunction, nervousness/agitation, discontinuation symptoms);

- pharmacokinetic interaction; and

- serotonergic syndrome.

SSRI neurochemistry

The neurochemistry of a typical SSRI is shown in Figure 9.14, but can be summarized as follows:

- selective 5-HT uptake blockade; and

- all SSRIs differ in chemical structures.

SSRI pharmacokinetics

SSRIs are rapidly absorbed and undergo hepatic metabolism. Some have active metabolites, but all are generally low in breast milk. Withdrawal effects are possible with drugs with a shorter half-life. The reported side-effects of SSRIs are presented in Figure 9.15.

SSRI efficacy

SSRIs are used for the acute treatment of episodes of depression. There is a 55–70% response rate after a 10–20 day delay in onset from starting treatment[1]. SSRIs are useful in preventing relapse, possibly because of good compliance.

Additionally, SSRIs are useful in the elderly with anxiety or OCD, those who are suicidal and possibly those with severe depression.

Prescription monitoring studies[13–15] show that older TCAs are commonly prescribed at lower than recommended doses, and for shorter than optimal periods. SSRIs are nearly always prescribed at doses proven to be effective and appear more likely to be prescribed for longer periods.

SSRIs may be preferable to older TCAs in the treatment of patients with a history of deliberate self-harm[1], as SSRI overdose is only rarely associated with medical complications.

Occasional case reports have described the emergence or worsening of suicidal thoughts during SSRI treatment, but analyses of pooled data from randomized controlled trials have shown that SSRIs are not associated with increases in suicidality[16,17] (see Figures 9.16 and 9.17).

At present, there is no direct evidence that patients prescribed SSRIs have a better outcome than those on TCAs[1]. The SSRIs are more expensive than older antidepressant drugs, but current pharmacoeconomic data do not favor initial treatment with one antidepressant over another[1]. The cost-effectiveness of SSRIs and TCAs in the treatment of depression in United Kingdom primary care is currently being evaluated (the University of Southampton 'Ahead' Study, supported by the Heath Technology Assessment Programme).

Discontinuation of SSRI treatment

Discontinuation symptoms may occur on abruptly stopping all classes of antidepressant drugs. The reported incidence varies widely, but symptoms are mild for most patients and usually resolve within 2 weeks. Comparative data are available for only the SSRIs, where paroxetine appears most likely, and fluoxetine least likely to be associated with discontinuation reactions[1]. Discontinuation symptoms appear less likely in shorter courses of treatment and if the drug dosage is tapered, but controlled evidence for tapering treatment is lacking. The March 2000 edition of the British National Formulary (BNF) states that abrupt withdrawal of an SSRI should be avoided. There is no consensus on the pharmacologic management of established SSRI discontinuation syndrome, but the results of a controlled study with SSRIs show that reinstatement of the original drug may relieve symptoms.

SEROTONIN–NOREPINEPHRINE REUPTAKE INHIBITORS

Examples of the SNRIs include venlafaxine and milnacipran (Figure 9.18).

Venlafaxine

Venlafaxine inhibits the presynaptic re-uptake of serotonin and NE, and to a much lesser extent dopamine (see Figure 9.19). Unlike TCAs, it has little or no affinity for adrenergic, cholinergic or histaminic receptors. It is effective in depressed patients in primary and secondary care settings, and in patients with generalized anxiety disorder (GAD).

A review of the findings of randomized controlled trials indicates that the short-term efficacy of venlafaxine is at least as good as that of the TCAs clomipramine and imipramine and the SSRIs paroxetine and fluoxetine[18]. In longer-term treatment, pooled analysis suggests that venlafaxine is efficacious in preventing relapse of depression[18]. A recent meta-analysis of the findings of comparator-controlled studies suggests that venlafaxine is significantly more efficacious than SSRIs in short-term treatment[19], and treatment with dual-acting drugs such as venlafaxine may be preferable to SSRI treatment in hospitalized depressed patients[1]. Venlafaxine has also been found efficacious in the treatment of GAD, in both short-term[20] and long-term treatment[21].

Venlafaxine appears to be tolerated as well as or better than clomipramine, dothiepin, imipramine, maprotiline and trazodone. In clinical trials, a rise in blood pressure was seen in some patients treated with venlafaxine, most often at doses above 200 mg per day (see Table 1).

The probability of clinically significant increases in blood pressure (rises greater than 15 mmHg, to a diastolic pressure greater than 105 mmHg), increases with dose, being 13% at doses above 300 mg per day[22]. Blood pressure should be monitored in those on doses above 200 mg per day, and venlafaxine should not be given to patients with hypertension. Discontinuation effects can occur when patients stop venlafaxine abruptly, particularly after daily doses of 150 mg or more: typically symptoms arise within 2 days, and resolve within a week of stopping treatment.

The reported side-effects of SNRIs are presented in Figure 9.20.

SELECTIVE NOREPINEPHRINE REUPTAKE INHIBITORS

Reboxetine is the typical example of the group of antidepressants termed the selective NERIs (see Figure 9.21).

Reboxetine

Reboxetine is a selective NERI, which has recently become available in a number of countries. It has little effect on 5-HT or dopamine re-uptake, does not inhibit MAO, and has low affinity for α-adrenergic and muscarinic receptors (see Figure 9.22).

In a series of randomized controlled trials, reboxetine has been found an efficacious antidepressant, in both short-term and long-term treatment. It has comparable efficacy to the TCAs imipramine and desipramine, and the SSRI fluoxetine[23]. Reboxetine may have certain advantages over fluoxetine, both in 'energizing' lethargic patients and in improving their social function[24]. Clinical experience has shown that reboxetine can be effective when patients have not responded to other antidepressants[25], and in combination treatment with an SSRI in partial responders to previous SSRI treatment[26]. Although reboxetine has proved efficacious in severely ill patients of younger and older age, it is not presently indicated for the treatment of depression in elderly patients. Recently presented data indicate that reboxetine is effective in the treatment of patients with panic disorder.

In an analysis of over 2600 patients included in clinical trials with reboxetine[27], it appeared generally well tolerated, the rate of discontinuation from treatment because of adverse events being similar to that with placebo. Dry mouth (27%), constipation (17%) and increased sweating (14%) were all significantly more frequent with reboxetine than with placebo, but were less common than with imipramine or desipramine. The frequency of adverse events with reboxetine (67%) is similar to that with fluoxetine (65%). Between 4% and 12% of patients, mainly men, develop urinary hesitancy with reboxetine, and the drug should not be prescribed to men with prostatic enlargement. A case report has described the development of urinary hesitancy with reboxetine, relieved by concomitant prescription of doxazosin. The profile of adverse events in clinical practice is similar to that in clinical trials, and those reactions reported to the Medicines Control Agency seem predictable, from knowledge of the pharmacologic properties of the drug.

Preliminary studies show that reboxetine does not inhibit the cytochrome P450 enzymes involved in the metabolism of other drugs, suggesting a low potential for drug–drug interactions[28]. However, reboxetine should be used cautiously when prescribed with drugs that are metabolized by CYP3A4 (e.g. antiarrhythmic drugs), and it should not be given with drugs that potently inhibit CYP3A4. In clinical trials, reboxetine did not appear to have any sustained effects on blood pressure, although up to 10% of patients may experience symptoms related to hypotension or tachycardia. Reboxetine should be used with caution in patients with cardiac disease, and in those taking antihypertensives.

Suicide attempts were infrequent in the clinical trials with reboxetine, occurring less often than with placebo, fluoxetine or imipramine. No deaths or serious sequelae following reboxetine overdose had been described by November 1998; the most common effects are sweating and tachycardia, but anxiety, postural hypotension and hypertension can also occur.

The side-effects of the NERIs are summarized in Figure 9.23.

Nefazodone

Nefazodone has a distinct pharmacologic profile, which includes moderate inhibition of the re-uptake of serotonin into presynaptic neurons and antagonism of postsynaptic 5-HT$_2$ receptors[29]. It is chemically related to trazodone (see Figure 9.24), but is a less potent antagonist at α_1-receptors (see Figure 9.25). Because of its blockade of 5-HT$_2$ receptors, it was anticipated that nefazodone would cause less treatment-emergent insomnia, anxiety and sexual dysfunction than SSRIs.

The efficacy of nefazodone in acute treatment of depression has been established in several double-blind placebo-controlled studies[30–32], and in a comparative study with paroxetine[33]. Treatment with nefazodone may offer some advantages over treatment with SSRIs, some studies showing less sleep disturbance[34], less increased anxiety[35] or treatment-emergent sexual dysfunction[36] with nefazodone. A recent study[37] found that continuing treatment with nefazodone was significantly better than switching to placebo, after an initial response to acute treatment.

One review[38] indicates that somnolence, nausea, dry mouth and dizziness are reported in around 5–10% of patients treated with nefazodone (see Figure 9.26), leading to dropout rates similar to those seen with fluoxetine or placebo, whereas another[39] estimates that these adverse events are more frequent, occurring in around 10–20% of subjects. Sexual dysfunction is reported only rarely during treatment, and nefazodone can be used to relieve sexual dysfunction caused by other antidepressants; however, like other antidepressants it has been implicated in the development of clitoral priapism[40]. Like the SSRIs, nefazodone can occasionally cause akathisia. Nefazodone appears less likely than trazodone to cause hypotension, because of reduced α_1 blocking properties[39]. A small proportion (2–3%) of patients develop visual 'trails' (usually after-images of moving objects) or 'shimmering' which can prove troublesome when driving.

Although nefazodone is a weak inhibitor of cytochrome $P450_{2D6}$, it causes potent inhibition of cytochrome $P450_{3A4}$, and so should not be given with terfenadine, astemizole, alprazolam, triazolam, cisapride or cyclosporin. Combination treatment with nefazodone and lithium appears generally well tolerated and safe. Nefazodone was possibly implicated in the development of sub-fulminant hepatic failure in a series of three patients, leading to suggestions that liver function tests should be performed before and during treatment.

Mirtazapine

Mirtazapine acts as an antagonist at pre-synaptic α_2-receptors and at postsynaptic 5-HT$_2$, 5-HT$_3$ and histamine H$_1$ receptors (see Figures 9.27 and 9.28). These complex actions result in enhanced serotonergic and noradrenergic neurotransmission across the synapses; the blockade of 5-HT$_2$ and 5-HT$_3$ receptors being responsible for a lower incidence of insomnia, sexual dysfunction and nausea, when compared to SSRIs[41].

A review of the findings of double-blind controlled treatment studies indicates that mirtazapine is at least as effective as reference TCA antidepressants such as amitriptyline or clomipramine[42]. Further studies indicate that mirtazapine may have an earlier onset of action than the SSRIs fluoxetine, citalopram and paroxetine, with similar rates of dropout due to adverse effects[43]. Like nefazodone, mirtazapine may have a particular role in the treatment of depressed patients troubled by insomnia or marked anxiety, or sexual dysfunction[44].

Mirtazapine has minimal anticholinergic, adrenergic or typical SSRI-type side-effects (see Figure 9.29). The only adverse events significantly more frequent with mirtazapine than with placebo are drowsiness (23% versus 14%), excessive sedation (19% versus 5%), dry mouth (25% versus 16%), increased appetite (11% versus 2%) and weight increase (10% versus 1%): by contrast, headache occurred significantly less often with mirtazapine (5% versus 10%)[45]. Typical SSRI-type adverse events, such as nausea, vomiting, diarrhea and insomnia are less frequent in mirtazapine-treated than in placebo-treated patients; unlike the SSRIs, mirtazapine does not appear to cause sexual dysfunction. Mirtazapine is better tolerated than amitriptyline, with significantly lower dropout rates due to adverse clinical experiences. Mirtazapine appears to have a low seizure-inducing potential, even though H$_1$-receptor antagonists are known to lower the seizure threshold.

Mirtazapine has minimal inhibitory effects on the cytochrome P450 metabolizing enzymes *in vitro*, sug-

gesting a low potential for drug–drug interactions. Mirtazapine appears to be safe when taken in overdose. Reversible white blood cell disorders (neutropenia and agranulocytosis) have been reported with mirtazapine, and treatment should be stopped and a blood count taken when fever, sore throat, stomatitis or other signs of infection occur.

OTHER DRUGS USED IN THE TREATMENT OF DEPRESSION

Trazodone

Trazodone blocks postsynaptic α_1-adrenoceptors, increases NE and 5-HT turnover (see Figures 9.30 and 9.31). It has antagonist actions at 5-HT$_2$ receptors, but its active metabolite *m*-chlorophenylpiperazine (*m*-CPP) is a 5-HT receptor agonist. Therefore the precise balance of effects on 5-HT receptors during treatment is difficult to determine. Trazodone has low cardiotoxicity and is less toxic in overdose than tricyclic antidepressants. Anticholinergic side-effects are also lower but there is an increased incidence of drowsiness and nausea (particularly if taken on an empty stomach). Side-effects are summarized in Figure 9.32.

A review of several placebo-controlled studies has shown that trazodone in doses of 150–600 mg is superior to placebo in the treatment of depressed patients[46]. It appears to have similar efficacy to imipramine. The major unwanted effect of trazodone is excessive sedation, which can result in significant cognitive impairment. Some patients experience postural hypotension due to its antagonism of α_1-adrenoceptors. The most serious side-effect of trazodone is priapism, which has an incidence of about 1 in 6000 male patients; sexual dysfunction is otherwise less troublesome than with many other antidepressant drugs.

Maprotiline

Maprotiline is a modified TCA (Figure 9.30) that is the most selective NERI among the TCAs, with little action on muscarinic or histamine receptors (see Figure 9.33). In comparative studies it appears to have comparable efficacy to that of other TCAs[47]. Unfortunately, it may precipitate seizures in patients predisposed to epilepsy and has a high incidence of seizures at doses above 200 mg. Therefore a maximum dose of 150 mg has been recommended. Like other TCAs it is potentially cardiotoxic in overdose. Reported side-effects are summarized in Figure 9.34. A long-term study found a higher rate of suicide attempts with maprotiline than with placebo[48].

Mianserin

Mianserin was the first truly atypical 'tetracyclic' antidepressant (Figure 9.35). It has a weak inhibitory effect on norepinephrine reuptake and is a potent antagonist at a number of 5-HT receptor subtypes (particularly 5-HT_{2A} and 5-HT_{2C} receptors). There is no antagonist effect at muscarinic cholinergic receptors. Figure 9.36 summarizes mianserin's mode of action.

Mianserin is a competitive antagonist at histamine H_1 receptors and α_1- and α_2-adrenoceptors. It can cause troublesome drowsiness, which is enhanced by alcohol, but has a good safety profile in overdose with low cardiotoxicity (Figure 9.37).

Controlled trials have shown that mianserin is superior to placebo in the management of depression, and comparable to imipramine and clomipramine[47]. The long-term efficacy of mianserin is not proven. The main adverse effects of mianserin are drowsiness, dizziness, weight gain, dyspepsia and nausea.

Cognitive impairment is more likely with mianserin than with SSRIs[49]. As with other tricyclics, mianserin increases the risk of seizures, and some patients may experience postural hypotension.

The most serious adverse effect of mianserin is the lowering of the white cell count, while fatal agranulocytosis has been reported. These are seen more commonly in the elderly. The BNF (4.3.1) recommends a full blood count every 4 weeks during the first 3 months of treatment with clinical monitoring continuing throughout treatment. Treatment should stop, and a full blood count be taken if any signs of infection develop (e.g. fever, sore throat or stomatitis). Other rare side-effects of mianserin include arthritis and hepatitis.

L-Tryptophan

L-Tryptophan is a naturally occurring amino acid and precursor to serotonin. It has a weak antidepressant effect, and is usually used as an adjunct for MAOIs and TCAs. Tryptophan deficiency causes a lowering of mood and tryptophan depletion has been shown to reverse antidepressant-induced remission from depression. Some preparations of L-tryptophan were associated with eosinophilia–myalgia syndrome (EMS) a potentially fatal connective tissue disease caused by a very high circulat-

ing eosinophil count with symptoms of muscle or joint pain, edema, skin sclerosis, peripheral neuropathy and fever (see Figure 9.38). Therefore in the UK it is only licensed for use by hospital specialists in patients with severe depression which has been continuous for more than 2 years. In addition there must have been adequate trials of a standard drug treatment, and it can be used only as an adjunct to other antidepressant medication. Patients' eosinophil levels must be closely monitored for signs and symptoms of EMS. The patient and prescriber must be registered with the Optimax Information and Clinical Support (OPTICS) Unit, with progress reported at 3 and 6 months, then 6-monthly. Other potential unwanted effects include sedation, myoclonus and serotonergic syndrome when combined with SSRIs.

Bupropion

Bupropion acts to increase dopaminergic neurotransmission. It has proven antidepressant effects, and may be especially helpful in the treatment of patients with bipolar depression. It has recently been licensed in the UK for use in smoking cessation. Most adverse effects arise from overstimulation of dopaminergic function, resulting in insomnia, agitation, nausea and weight loss (see Figure 9.39). It has few, if any, sedative, anticholingergic, hypotensive or cardiotoxic properties although psychosis can occur occasionally. There is also an increased risk of seizures. Bupropion should not be coadministered with MAOIs or dopamine precursors or agonists (e.g. levodopa and other antiparkinsonian drugs).

ANTIDEPRESSANT DRUG TREATMENT OF BEREAVEMENT-RELATED PROBLEMS

Depressive symptoms are frequently seen as a normal part of the grieving process and some clinicians believe that the treatment of the symptoms of bereavement-related depression may interfere with the normal grieving process, also for some doctors the medicalization of grief is a contentious issue. However, in primary care the recognition and treatment of depressive disorders remains poor and therefore it is not uprising that bereavement-related depression tends to be untreated. Zisook and colleagues[50] found 83% of bereaved spouses who met criteria for major depressive syndrome received no antidepressant medication. However, the authors suggested that when there is a prolonged grief reaction of more than 6 months, which meets the criteria for major or minor depressive disorders, then these should be diagnosed and treated as mood disorders.

Several antidepressants have been studied in bereaved people. In a small-scale open trial, Pasternak and coworkers[51] found nortriptyline to be effective in treating people with bereavement-related depression in late life. Zygmont and associates[52] carried out an open-trial pilot study of paroxetine for symptoms of traumatic grief, compared with the effects of nortriptyline in an archival contrast group, from an ongoing separate study. Fifteen mixed bereaved people were treated with paroxetine which began at a median of 17 months postbereavement (range 6–139 months). In addition each person received psychotherapy tailored for traumatic grief. The results from the paroxetine group were a 53% decrease in the level of traumatic grief symptoms, and a 54% decrease in depressive symptoms as measured by the Hamilton Rating Scale for Depression (HAM-D). Paroxetine was comparable to nortriptyline, although the authors favored the use of paroxetine for traumatic grief, owing to the greater safety in overdose.

Reynolds and colleagues[53] carried out a placebo controlled study of nortriptyline alone, nortriptyline combined with interpersonal psychotherapy, placebo alone and combined with interpersonal psychotherapy. Nortriptyline was superior to placebo, although there was no effect found from interpersonal psychotherapy. One interesting finding was that, although nortriptyline was efficacious in treating depressive symptoms, it had no effect on the intensity of grief (measured by the Texas Revised Inventory of Grief). The authors offered two theoretical explanations: first, that depressive symptoms may represent biological dysregulation (e.g. sleep and appetitive disturbances), which are more amenable to pharmacologic intervention; and second, that grief intensity may represent other factors such as unresolved problems of loss and difficulty in performing role transition tasks. Alternatively they suggested that persistent grief (e.g. preoccupation with the memories) may not be abnormal or pathologic.

There is little support for prescribing antidepressant drugs to bereaved people without bereavement-related problems. However, the use is advocated for those with bereavement-related depression and anxiety, and traumatic grief.

The SSRIs have a number of advantages as the choice of therapy for bereavement-related depression, as they have a broad spectrum of efficacy in the treatment of depressive disorders and anxiety disorders (panic disorder, OCD, social phobia and post-traumatic stress disorder) that are seen in bereavement. In addition they are relatively safe in overdose. Unlike TCAs, SSRIs have no carditoxicity in overdose, and the increased risk of death from cardiovascular disease within the first 6 months of bereavement is an important variable to consider.

USE OF COMPLEMENTARY MEDICINES

Many patients describe some benefit from complementary approaches such as instruction in the Alexander technique or meditation, although 'scientific' evidence for the efficacy of these approaches is lacking. In certain countries, many depressed patients are treated with St John's Wort (*Hypericum perforatum*), a 'herbal' remedy; in other areas, it is used in a wide range of conditions, including premenstrual syndrome, bereavement, insomnia and stress. A review of clinical trials has suggested that *H. perforatum* is more efficacious than placebo in the treatment of patients with depression of mild or moderate intensity. Many patients are attracted to the preparation because of its 'natural' origins and presumed safety, although different formulations vary in the bioavailability of the active principle (which has some SSRI-like properties).

St John's Wort

St John's Wort or *H. perforatum* is a plant native to Europe, used for centuries as a herbal remedy for its wound healing, antiviral, anti-inflammatory, sedative and antidepressant properties[54,55]. It can be taken in a variety of ways, preferably as tablets containing the dried alcoholic extract of the herb, standardized to provide a given amount of one of the constituents, usually hypericin. There are many other compounds present in *H. perforatum* extract, including naphtodianthrons, flavenoids, xanthones and bioflavenoids, which probably exert their effects via different mechanisms[56]. Extracts are standardized to only one component, resulting in heterogeneity between brands; to minimize this, many treatment studies use the LI160 extract.

The mode of action of St John's Wort is poorly understood, but may depend on alterations in neurotransmitter concentrations and receptor density at postsynaptic neurones[57]. It inhibits the re-uptake of 5-HT, dopamine and norepinephrine[57,58], causes stimulation of GABA receptors and is a weak MAOI[58]. The results of two meta-analyses suggest that around 60–70% of patients with mild–moderate depression respond to treatment[56,57]. One of these[56] concluded that *H. perforatum* extract was significantly more effective than placebo and similarly effective to conventional antidepressant medication. More recent studies have also found *H. perforatum* to be effective, including a three-arm study comparing *H. perforatum* (1050 mg extract/day), imipramine (100 mg/day) and placebo[59]. *H. perforatum* has also been found useful in the treatment of seasonal affective disorder (SAD)[60].

H. perforatum use may result in the induction of various drug-metabolizing systems including cytochrome P450 3A4, 1A2, 2C9 and P-glycoprotein (a transport protein)[58]. This can cause decreased efficacy or plasma concentrations of a number of drugs, including warfarin, oral contraceptives, anticonvulsants, digoxin, cyclosporin, theophylline, and HIV protease and non-nucleoside reverse transcriptase inhibitors.

H. perforatum is generally well tolerated, a recent review finding an incidence of adverse effects similar to that for placebo[61]. Side-effects are usually mild-to-moderate and transient, and include gastrointestinal disturbance, restlessness, dizziness, fatigue, dry mouth and (rarely) allergic reactions[57,58,61]. Photosensitivity is very rare at therapeutic doses, it being estimated that a dose 30–50 times the recommended amount would be required to cause severe phototoxic reactions[61].

TREATMENT OF COEXISTING ANXIETY DISORDERS

Managing patients with generalized anxiety disorder

Many features of GAD are similar to those of depression. To differentiate GAD from depressive illness patients should be questioned about symptoms such as loss of interest and pleasure, loss of appetite and weight, diurnal variation in mood and early morning waking. Patients who present with no obvious psychologic explanation or episodic symptoms without apparent cause should be examined for thyrotoxicosis, pheochromocytoma and hypoglycemia.

Caffeine is best avoided by patients with GAD, as there is some evidence of abnormal sensitivity in some patients[62]. It is useful for patients to identify potential causes of anxiety and psychologic therapies to help the patient develop strategies for anxiety management (e.g. cognitive–behavior therapy (CBT), problem-solving techniques).

Drug treatment of GAD

Benzodiazepines can be effective in providing short-term relief, but they can cause troublesome sedation and carry a long-term risk of dependence. They are best prescribed when the patient has particularly distressing or disabling anxiety symptoms, for short treatment courses only. Drugs that have proven efficacy in randomized controlled trials include buspirone (a partial agonist of the serotonin 5-HT$_{1A}$ receptor), some TCAs (e.g. imipramine), paroxetine, trazodone and the SNRI venlafaxine. The antipsychotic drug trifluoperazine is sometimes effective in reducing anxiety but is associated with a number of long-term side-effects[63].

The treatment options for GAD are summarized in Figure 9.40.

Managing patients with panic disorder and agoraphobia

There are numerous medical conditions that produce panic-like symptoms and these should be considered and excluded before treatment of panic disorder. These medical conditions include other mental disorders (e.g. schizophrenia, mood disorder or somatoform disorder), alcohol and drug withdrawal, caffeinism, hyperthyroidism, hyperparathyroidism, hypoglycemia, pheochromocytoma, cardiac arrhythmias, labyrinthitis and temporal lobe epilepsy.

Owing to the high rates of comorbid depression, it is important to treat the symptoms of both anxiety and depression. The SSRIs paroxetine and citalopram are licensed in the UK as treatments for panic disorder, and SSRIs have been recommended as drugs of first choice. A meta-analysis of 27 placebo-controlled randomized controlled trials concluded that treatment with SSRIs was more effective than treatment with either imipramine or alprazolam[64]. A consensus statement on panic disorder from the International Consensus Group on Depression and Anxiety recommends treatment with SSRIs and suggests a long-term treatment period of 12–24 months, which should be discontinued slowly over 4–6 months[65]. Some patients experience a transient worsening of panic in the first few weeks of treatment and all should be warned about this potential side-effect. Other antidepressant drugs found to be effective include certain TCAs (imipramine, clomipramine and lofepramine).

High-potency benzodiazepines (e.g. alprazolam, clonazepam and lorazepam) are effective in many patients, but should be reserved for severely ill patients and only used for short-term treatment. MAOIs (e.g. phenelzine) have been found to be effective in the treatment of panic disorders, but tend to be used less frequently, owing to the need for dietary restrictions and side-effects. The RIMAs (e.g. moclobemide), although not licensed for the treatment of panic, demonstrate potential efficacy and have the benefits of minimum dietary restriction.

Behavior therapy (e.g. exposure to phobic situation and training in coping with panic attacks) and cognitive therapy are also beneficial in many patients.

MANAGING PATIENTS WITH SPECIFIC (ISOLATED) PHOBIAS

Traditionally, patients with specific phobias are treated by behavior therapy using cognitive techniques, such as exposure behavior therapy (e.g. fear of flying courses run by the large airline companies). Antidepressant drugs can be used in patients with persistent and disabling specific phobias that have proven resistant to behavioral treatments.

MANAGEMENT OF SOCIAL PHOBIA

SSRIs are recommended as first-line pharmacologic therapy, and treatment is suggested for at least 12 months[66]. Several SSRIs have been found efficacious in the short-term treatment of patients with social phobia,

the most studied drugs being paroxetine and sertraline. Others drugs include MAOIs (e.g. penelzine) and the RIMA moclobemide. There is no published good evidence for the efficacy of TCAs or β-blockers in generalized social phobia, and although certain benzodiazepines have been found efficacious in randomized controlled trials, the same cautions apply against their use as do in the treatment of panic disorder. Table 2 presents the pharmacologic treatment options that have undergone treatment studies. Effective psychologic therapies include individual cognitive restructuring, coupled with exposure therapy and group CBT.

MANAGEMENT OF POST-TRAUMATIC STRESS DISORDER

The first step in the management of post-traumatic stress disorder (PTSD) is to distinguish between the acute and chronic conditions, and assess the predominant features. The first 3 months after the incident are critical and not everyone with acute PTSD develops the chronic form. There are three main phases of management, namely acute symptom stabilization (4–12 weeks), maintenance therapy (12 months) and discontinuation.

The acute stage of treatment is aimed to reduce initial distress by supportive and empathic listening aimed at reducing feelings of helplessness and guilt. The provision of information related to disability, compensation

Table 2 Pharmacologic treatment options for social phobia that have undergone treatment studies[67]

Class of drug	Examples (generic name)	Comments
Beta-blockers	Atenolol	Not recommended as a treatment option
Benzodiazepines	Alprazolam, Clonazepam, Bromazepam	Best avoided when there is evidence of comorbidity with alcohol abuse. May cause excessive sedation
Tricyclic antidepressants	Imipramine	Not recommended as a treatment option
Non-selective monoamine oxidase inhibitors (MAOIs)	Phenelzine	Evidence of efficacy. Patient must adhere to strict tyramine-free diet
Reversible inhibitors of monoamine oxidase type A (RIMAs)	Moclobemide (also Brofaromine)	Evidence of efficacy. Some possible restriction on diet
Selective serotonin reuptake inhibitors (SSRIs)	Citalopram Fluoxetine Fluvoxamine Sertraline Paroxetine	Recommended as first-line therapy in the pharmacologic treatment of social anxiety disorder Paroxetine, fluvoxamine and sertraline have demonstrated safety, efficacy and tolerability in double-blind, placebo-controlled treatment studies
Novel antidepressant	Nefazodone	Evidence of efficacy from case reports and open trials
Serotonin/norepinephrine reuptake inhibitor (SNRI)	Venlafaxine	Evidence of efficacy from case reports and open trials
Anticonvulsants	Gabapentin, Pregabalin	Efficacious in randomized controlled trials Poor tolerability at higher doses

and community support groups can help people to take control and 'fight back'. Benzodiazepines may be useful for short-term treatment to reduce arousal and psychologic repression of the traumatic event, but are not recommended for long-term use.

Overall, SSRIs are probably the drug treatment of choice for PTSD, evidenced by randomized controlled trials investigating fluoxetine, paroxetine and sertraline[68]. Some TCAs (e.g. amitriptyline, imipramine) produce significant improvement, but are less effective than SSRIs.

The RIMA brofaromine has also demonstrated some efficacy, as has the MAOI phenelzine[69]. However, caution is advised with MAOIs due to the high comorbidity with alcohol and drug abuse in patients with PTSD, as drug interactions with MAOIs can be dangerous. The most effective psychologic treatment is CBT.

MANAGEMENT OF OBSESSIVE–COMPULSIVE DISORDER

Most patients with OCD require a combination of management approaches, including patient education, drug treatment with SSRIs or clomipramine and cognitive behavioral techniques. The SSRIs are clearly efficacious in patients with OCD, both in short- and long-term treatment. The efficacy of SSRIs or clomipramine is not dependent upon the presence of co-existing depressive symptoms. An emerging amount of literature supports the use of SSRIs in the treatment of children and adolescents with OCD, as well as in adults[70].

OCD is usually a chronic disorder, waxing and waning in severity over time, and the magnitude of change during acute treatment studies can therefore be rather disappointing.

The relative efficacy and tolerability of clomipramine and the SSRIs in the management of patients with OCD has been discussed extensively[70]. Although there are occasional studies indicating that an SSRI is more efficacious than clomipramine, systematic reviews and meta-analyses have shown that treatment with clomipramine is marginally, but significantly, more effective than treatment with SSRIs[71–73]. In turn, SSRIs are more effective than drugs that do not have serotonin re-uptake inhibition as part of their mechanism of action. The main advantage for SSRIs is their improved tolerability profile compared to clomipramine[70], which suggests that SSRIs should be considered a first-line pharmacologic treatment for patients with OCD, clomipramine being reserved for those patients who do not show signs of improvement with fluvoxamine, fluoxetine, paroxetine or sertraline.

LITHIUM AND OTHER MOOD-STABILIZING DRUGS

The acute treatment of mania usually involves lithium, valproate compounds and antipsychotic drugs, sometimes in combination. Antipsychotic drugs may have an earlier onset of action than lithium, but are less well tolerated. Lithium and valproate are more often used as prophylactic treatments, in an attempt to reduce the risk of future manic or depressive episodes.

Lithium

Randomized controlled trials of lithium treatment have shown that it is effective in 60–90% of acutely ill patients with manic episodes, and in up to 80% of patients when used in the long-term prophylaxis of bipolar affective disorder[74]. Lithium is also effective in the prophylaxis of recurrent unipolar depressive disorder, though not as effective as treatment with antidepressant drugs. It is disappointing that the good results seen with lithium in randomized controlled trials are often not replicated in the different setting of routine clinical practice, where lithium treatment is not always undertaken in the optimal fashion (see Figure 9.41).

Treatment can be improved through setting up specialized lithium clinics and through setting up local protocols for care. The best results in bipolar illness are seen when treatment is good, there is a family history of bipolar illness and when episodes of mania are followed by depression. Poorer results are seen in rapid cycling illness, in patients with comorbid substance abuse and when paranoid features are present.

When prescribed rationally and taken regularly, lithium can alter the course of bipolar affective disorder. There is also some evidence that lithium treatment can reduce the overall mortality associated with bipolar illness and reduce suicide rates. Conversely, many patients will derive little benefit from lithium treatment, only experiencing side-effects such as thirst, polyuria, tremor and weight gain. Lithium treatment can also cause a mild impairment of attention and memory, worsen or precipitate skin problems and cause a leukocytosis. Hypothyroidism and a non-toxic goiter can occur in around 5% of patients, and a further 5–10% of patients may experience impaired renal tubular function whilst undergoing long-term treatment. Use during pregnancy should be avoided whenever possible, as teratogenic effects may be seen in up to 11% of births, cardiovascular malformations being among the more common abnormalities. Figure 9.42 summarizes the side-effects of lithium.

Lithium levels can increase during concomitant treatment with diuretics, nonsteroidal anti-inflammatory drugs and angiotensin-converting enzyme inhibitors. Central nervous system toxicity can be worsened by antidepressants, antipsychotics, some antihypertensives and, possibly, some general anesthetics.

Lithium toxicity can occur insidiously, although signs of toxicity usually appear when levels rise above 1.3 mmol/l[74]. At first, patients become troubled by worsening tremor, nausea and vomiting. Later signs include drowsiness, disorientation, dysarthria, convulsions and coma. Pulmonary complications and cardiac effects can lead to death. Treatment of established lithium toxicity involves admission, rehydration and anticonvulsants; hemodialysis may be required when lithium levels are greater than 3.0 mmol/l, in comatose patients and when simpler measures have not improved matters within 24 h[74].

Prior to starting lithium treatment, the degree of affective morbidity should be established, the need for long-term treatment should be discussed, the patient should be weighed, blood tests should be performed for renal and thyroid function and pregnancy tests should be performed in women of childbearing potential. A starting dose of around 600 mg should be used in healthy young adults, determining lithium levels after 5–7 days[74]. The target for these levels should be 0.5–1.0 mmol/l.

Monitoring patients during lithium treatment is best done within a mood disorders clinic so that affective symptoms can be monitored conscientiously and sleep disturbance can be treated. The attempt should be made to give all the daily dose of lithium at night, and the patient should be asked about adherence at each visit.

The use of additional psychotropic drugs is recommended if response is partial. Lithium level should be assessed every 3 months, and an estimate of renal and thyroid function should be made every 6 months. Lithium should be discontinued slowly.

Anticonvulsants

Treatment with an anticonvulsant may be effective in patients with rapid cycling bipolar illness, in those with mixed affective episodes and when lithium has been only partially helpful. Both carbamazepine (Figure 9.43) and valproate compounds have been found efficacious in the acute treatment of mania, and there is some evidence of benefit in the prophylaxis of bipolar illness[75]. Both lamotrigine and topiramate are being evaluated in extensive clinical trial programs in the area of bipolar illness.

Sodium valproate was first used in the treatment of primary generalized epilepsy, generalized absences and myoclonic seizures. It is now also used in patients with treatment-refractory mania and long-term treatment in rapid cycling illness, particularly in nonpsychotic patients. Recent controlled trials indicate that valproate compounds may prevent new episodes of affective illness[76]. The adverse effects of treatment include nausea, vomiting and hair loss. Blood dyscrasias and hepatotoxicity can also occur, and full blood tests and liver function tests should be performed regularly during treatment. Valproate can interact with certain antidepressant and antipsychotic drugs, and antimalarials. Like lithium, valproate is also potentially teratogenic and can cause abnormalities of the heart, neural tube, lip and palate. Because of this, it should be used with great caution during pregnancy.

The adverse effects of carbamazepine include headache, drowsiness, nausea and vomiting. It can cause skin rashes, blood dyscrasias and hepatic problems, including hepatitis and cholestatic jaundice. It can induce the metabolism of anticoagulants and certain antidepressant and antipsychotic drugs, steroids and oral contraceptives. Carbamazepine can also exert teratogenic effects, possibly through causing iatrogenic folate deficiency. Figure 9.44 summarizes the side-effects of the anticonvulsants.

REFERENCES

1. Anderson IM, Nutt DJ, Deakin JFW. Evidence-based guidelines for treating depressive illness with antidepressants: a revision of the 1993 British Association for Psychopharmacology guidelines. *J Psychopharmacol* 2000;14:3–20

2. Baldwin DS, Rudge SE. Moclobemide – a reversible inhibitor of monoamine oxidase type A. *Br J Hosp Med* 1993;49:497–9

3. Priest RG, Schmid-Burgk W. Moclobemide in the treatment of depression. *Rev Contemp Pharmacother* 1994;5:35–43

4. Angst J, Johnson FN. Moclobemide in special sub-groups of depression. *Rev Contemp Pharmacother* 1994;5:45–53

5. Versiani M, Nardi AE, Mundim FD, Alves AB, Liebowitz MR, Amrein R. Pharmacotherapy of social phobia. A controlled study with moclobemide and phenelzine. *Br J Psychiatry* 1992;161:353–60

6. The International Multicenter Clinical Trial Group on Moclobemide in Social Phobia. Moclobemide in social phobia. A double-blind, placebo-controlled clinical study. *Eur Arch Psychiatry Clin Neurosci* 1997;247:71–80

7. Nutt D, Baldwin DS, Beaumont G, *et al*. Guidelines for the management of social phobia/social anxiety disorder. *Prim Care Psychiatry* 1999;5:147–55

8. Dingemanse J, Wood N, Guentert T, Oie S, Ouwerkerk M, Amrein R. Clinical pharmacology of moclobemide during chronic administration of high doses to healthy subjects. *Psychopharmacology (Berl)* 1998;140:164–72

9. Dingemanse J, Guentert T, Gieschke R, Stabl M. Modification of the cardiovascular effects of ephedrine by the reversible monoamine oxidase A-inhibitor moclobemide. *J Cardiovasc Pharmacol* 1996;28:856–61

10. Song F, Freemantle N, Sheldon TA, *et al*. Selective serotonin reuptake inhibitors: meta-analysis of efficacy and acceptability. *Br Med J* 1993;306:683–7

11. Anderson IM. Lessons to be learnt from meta-analyses of newer versus older antidepressants. *Adv Psychiatric Treat* 1997;3:58–63

12. Geddes JR, Freemantle N, Mason J, *et al*. SSRIs versus alternative antidepressants in depressive disorder (Cochrane Review). In: The Cochrane Library, issue 4. Oxford, UK: Update Software, 1999

13. Rosholm JU, Gram LF, Isacsson G, *et al*. Changes in the pattern of antidepressant use upon the introduction of the new antidepressants: a prescription database study. *Eur J Clin Pharmacol* 1997;52:205–9

14. Donoghue J. Sub-optimal use of tricyclic antidepressants in primary care. *Acta Psych Scand* 1998;98:429–31

15. Dunn RL, Donoghue JM, Ozminkowski RJ, *et al*. Longitudinal patterns of antidepressant prescribing in primary care in the UK: comparison with treatment guidelines. *J Psychopharmacol* 1999;13:136–43

16. Beasley CM, Dornseif BE, Bosomworth JC, *et al*. Fluoxetine and suicide: a meta-analysis of controlled trials of treatment for depression. *Br Med J* 1991;303:685–92

17. Montgomery SA, Dunner DL, Dunbar GC. Reduction of suicidal thoughts with paroxetine in comparison with reference antidepressants and placebo. *Eur Neuropsychopharmacol* 1995;5:5–13

18. Burnett FE, Dinan TG. The clinical efficacy of venlafaxine in the treatment of depression. *Rev Contemp Pharmacother* 1998;9:303–20

19. Thase ME, Entsuah AR, Rudolph RL. Remission rates during treatment with venlafaxine or selective serotonin reuptake inhibitors. *Br J Psychiatry* 2001;178:234–41

20. Davidson JRT, DuPont RL, Hedges D, *et al*. Efficacy, safety, and tolerability of venlafaxine extended release and buspirone in outpatients with generalized anxiety disorder. *J Clin Psychiatry* 1999;60:528–30

21. Gelenberg AJ, Lydiard RB, Rudolph RL, *et al*. Efficacy of venlafaxine extended-release capsules in nondepressed outpatients with generalized anxiety disorder. *JAMA* 2000;283:3082–8

22. Rudolph RL, Derivan AT. The safety and tolerability of venlafaxine hydrochloride: analysis of the clinical trials database. *J Clin Psychopharmacol* 1996;16(suppl 2):54s–9s

23. De Maio D, Johnson FN. The clinical efficacy of reboxetine in the treatment of depression. *Rev Contemp Pharmacother* 2000;11:303–20

24. Healy D. Reboxetine, fluoxetine and social functioning as an outcome measure in clinical trials: implications. *Primary Care Psychiatry* 1998;4:81–9

25. Argyropoulos SV, Wheeler A, Nutt DJ. A case of reversal of treatment-resistant depression after almost 30 years of symptoms. *Int J Psychiatry Clin Pract* 1999;3:289–91

26. Baldwin DS, Hawley CJ, Szabadi E, *et al*. Reboxetine in the treatment of depression: early clinical experience in the UK. *Int J Psychiatry Clin Pract* 1998;2:195–201

27. Baldwin DS, Buis C, Carabal E. Tolerability and safety of reboxetine. *Rev Contemp Pharmacother* 2000;11:321–30

28. Dostert P, Benedetti MS, Poggesi I. Review of the pharmacokinetics and metabolism of reboxetine, a selective noradrenaline reuptake inhibitor. *Eur Neuropsychopharmacol* 1997;7 (suppl 1):s23–35

29. Eison AS, Eison MS, Torrente JR, *et al*. Nefazodone: preclinical pharmacology of a new antidepressant. *Psychopharmacology (Berl)* 1990;26:311–15

30. Cohn CK, Robinson DS, Roberts DL, *et al*. Responders to antidepressant drug treatment: a study comparing nefazodone, imipramine and placebo in patients with major depression. *J Clin Psychiatry* 1996;57 (suppl 2):2–18

31. Fontaine R, Ontiveros A, Elie R, *et al*. A double-blind comparison of nefazodone, imipramine and placebo in major depression. *J Clin Psychiatry* 1994;55:234–41

32. Rickels K, Schweizer E, Clary C, *et al*. Nefazodone and imipramine in major depression : a placebo-controlled trial. *Br J Psychiatry* 1994;164:802–5

33. Baldwin DS, Hawley CJ, Abed RT, *et al*. A multicenter double-blind comparison of nefazodone and paroxetine in the treatment of outpatients with moderate-to-severe depression. *J Clin Psychiatry* 1996;57 (suppl 2):46–52

34. Armitage R, Rush J, Trivedi M, *et al*. The effects of nefazodone on sleep architecture in depression. *Neuropsychopharmacology* 1994;10:123–7

35. Zajecka JM. The effect of nefazodone on comorbid anxiety symptoms associated with depression: experience in family practice and psychiatric outpatient settings. *J Clin Psychiatry* 1996;57 (suppl 2):10–14

36. Feiger A, Kiev A, Shrivastava RK, *et al*. Nefazodone versus sertraline in outpatients with major depression: focus on efficacy, tolerability and effects on sexual function and satisfaction. *J Clin Psychiatry* 1996;57 (suppl 2):53–62

37. Feiger AD, Bielski RJ, Bremner J, *et al*. Double-blind, placebo-substitution study of nefazodone in the prevention of relapse during continuation treatment of outpatients with major depression. *Int J Clin Psychopharmacol* 1999;14:19–28

38. Preskorn SH. Comparison of the tolerability of bupropion, fluoxetine, imipramine, nefazodone, paroxetine, sertraline, and venlafaxine. *J Clin Psychiatry* 1995;56 (suppl 6):12–21

39. Robinson DS, Roberts DL, Smith JM, *et al*. The safety profile of nefazodone. *J Clin Psychiatry* 1996;57 (suppl 2):31–8

40. Brodie-Meijer CCE, Diemont WL, Buijs PJ. Nefazodone-induced clitoral priapism. *Int Clin Psychopharmacol* 1999;14:257–8

41. Westenberg HGM. Pharmacology of antidepressants: selectivity or multiplicity? *J Clin Psychiatry* 1999;60 (suppl 17):4–8

42. Kasper S. Clinical efficacy of mirtazapine: a review of meta-analyses of pooled data. *Int J Clin Psychopharmacol* 1995;10:25–35

43. Thompson C. Mirtazapine versus selective serotonin reuptake inhibitors. *J Clin Psychiatry* 1999;60 (suppl 17):18–22

44. Baldwin DS, Thomas SC, Birtwistle J. Effects of antidepressant drugs on sexual function. *Int J Psychiatry Clin Pract* 1997;1:47–58

45. Montgomery S-A. Safety of mirtazapine: a review. *Int Clin Psychopharmacol* 1995;10 (suppl):437–45

46. Schatzberg AF. Trazodone: a 5-year review of antidepressant efficacy. *Psychopathology* 1987;20 (suppl 1):48–56

47. Anderson IM. Meta-analytical studies on new antidepressants. *Br Med Bull* 2001;57:161–78

48. Rouillon F, Phillips R, Serrurier D, Ansart E, Gerard MJ. Recurrence of unipolar depression and efficacy of maprotiline [in French]. *Encephale* 1989;15:527–34

49. Knegtering H, Eijck M, Huijsman A. Effects of antidepressants on cognitive functioning of elderly patients. A review. *Drugs Aging* 1994;5:192–9

50. Zisook S, Shuchter SR, Sledge PA, Paulus M, Judd LL. The spectrum of depressive phenomena after spousal bereavement. *J Clin Psychiatry* 1994;55 (suppl):29–36

51. Pasternak RE, Reynolds CF III, Schlernitzauer M, *et al*. Acute open-trial nortriptyline therapy of bereavement-related depression in late life. *J Clin Psychiatry* 1991;52:307–10

52. Zygmont M, Prigerson HG, Houck PR, *et al*. A post hoc comparison of paroxetine and nortriptyline for symptoms of traumatic grief. *J Clin Psychiatry* 1998;59:241–5

53. Reynolds CF III, Miller MD, Pasternak RE, *et al*. Treatment of bereavement-related major depressive episodes in later life: a controlled study of acute and continuation treatment with nortriptyline and interpersonal psychotherapy. *Am J Psychiatry* 1999;156:202–8

54. Barnes J, Anderson LA, Phillipson JD. St John's wort (*Hypericum perforatum* L.): a review of its chemistry, pharmacology and clinical properties. *J Pharmacy Pharmacol* 2001;53:583–600

55. Linde K, Mulrow CD. St John's wort for depression. *Cochrane Database Syst Rev* 2000;2:CD000448

56. Nahrstedt A, Butterweck V. Biologically active and other chemical constituents of the herb *Hypericum perforatum* L. *Pharmacopsychiatry* 1997;30:129–34

57. Nathan PJ. *Hypericum perforatum* (St John's Wort): a non-selective reuptake inhibitor? A review of the recent advances in its pharmacology. *J Psychopharmacol* 2001;15:47–54

58. Kientsch U, Burgi S, Ruedeberg C, Probst S, Honegger UE. St. John's wort extract Ze 117 (*Hypericum perforatum*) inhibits norepinephrine and serotonin uptake into rat brain slices and reduces β-adrenoceptor numbers on cultured rat brain cells. *Pharmacopsychiatry* 2001;34 (suppl 1):s56–60

59. Philipp M, Kohnen R, Hiller K-O. Hypericum extract versus imipramine or placebo in patients with moderate depression: randomised multicentre study of treatment for eight weeks. *Br Med J* 1999;319:1534–8

60. Wheatley D. Hypericum in seasonal affective disorder (SAD). *Curr Med Res Opin* 1999;15:33–7

61. Ernst E, Rand JI, Barnes J, Stevinson C. Adverse effects profile of the herbal antidepressant St. John's wort (*Hypericum perforatum* L.). *Eur J Clin Pharmacol* 1998;54:589–94

62. Bruce M, Scott N, Shine P, Lader M. Anxiogenic effects of caffeine in patients with anxiety disorders. *Arch Gen Psychiatry* 1992;49:867–9

63. Mendels J, Krajewski TF, Huffer V, *et al*. Effective short-term treatment of generalized anxiety disorder with trifluoperazine. *J Clin Psychiatry* 1986;47:170–4

64. Boyer W. Serotonin uptake inhibitors are superior to imipramine and alprazolam in alleviating panic attacks: a meta-analysis. *Int J Clin Psychopharmacol* 1995;10:45–9

65. Ballenger JC, Davidson JR, Lecrubier Y, *et al*. Consensus statement on panic disorder from the International Consensus Group on Depression and Anxiety. *J Clin Psychiatry* 1998;59 (Suppl 8):47–54

66. Ballenger JC, Davidson JR, Lecrubier Y, *et al*. Consensus statement on social anxiety disorder from the International Consensus Group on Depression and Anxiety. *J Clin Psychiatry* 1998;59 (suppl 17):54–6

67. Baldwin D. *La Fobia Sociale. Una Questione di Salute Pubblica?*. Rome: Il Pensiero Scientifica Editore, 2000

68. Davidson JRT, Connor KM. Serotonin and serotonergic drugs in post-traumatic stress disorder. In: Montgomery SA, den Boer JA, eds. *SSRIs in Depression and Anxiety. Perspectives in Psychiatry*, Volume 8. Chichester, UK: John Wiley, 2001:175–91

69. Baker DG, Diamond BI, Gillette G, *et al*. A double-blind, ran-

domized, placebo-controlled, multi-center study of bro-faromine in the treatment of post-traumatic stress disorder. *Psychopharmacology (Berl)* 1995;122:386–9

70. Montgomery SA. SSRIs in obsessive–compulsive disorder. In: Montgomery SA, den Boer JA, eds. *SSRIs in Depression and Anxiety. Perspectives in Psychiatry*, Volume 8. Chichester, UK: John Wiley, 2001:151–74

71. Cox BJ, Swinson RP, Morrison B, Lee PS. Clomipramine, fluoxetine, and behavior therapy in the treatment of obsessive-compulsive disorder: a meta-analysis. *J Behav Ther Exp Psychiatry* 1993;24:149–53

72. Piccinelli M, Pini S, Bellantuono C, Wilkinson G. Efficacy of drug treatment in obsessive-compulsive disorder. A meta-analytic review. *Br J Psychiatry* 1995;166:424–43

73. Stein DJ, Spadaccini E, Hollander E. Meta-analysis of pharmacotherapy trials for obsessive-compulsive disorder. *Int Clin Psychopharmacol* 1995;10:11–18

74. Ferrier IN, Tyrer SP, Bell AJ. Lithium therapy. *Adv Psychiatr Treat* 1995;1:102–10

75. Ferrier IN. Developments in mood stabilisers. *Br Med Bull* 2001;57:179–92

76. Bowden CL, Calabrese JR, McElroy SL, *et al.* A randomized, placebo-controlled 12-month trial of divalproex and lithium in treatment of outpatients with bipolar I disorder. Divalproex Maintenance Study Group. *Arch Gen Psychiatry* 2000;57:481–9

BIBLIOGRAPHY

Donoghue JM. The prescribing of antidepressants in general practice: the use of PACT data (brief report). *Postgrad Med J* 1994;70 (suppl 2):S23–4

Donoghue JM, Tylee A. The treatment of depression: prescribing patterns of antidepressants in primary care in the UK. *Br J Psychiatry* 1996;168:164–8

MacDonald TM, McMahon AD, Reid IC, Fenton GW, McDevitt DG. Antidepressant drug use in primary care: a record linkage study in Tayside, Scotland. *Br Med J* 1996;313:860–1

CHAPTER 10

Physical treatments for depression

ELECTROCONVULSIVE THERAPY

Electroconvulsive therapy (ECT) involves the induction of a brief seizure induced by passing an electrical current across a patient's brain following the administration of a general anesthetic and a muscle relaxant. ECT has a potent antidepressant effect, which has an earlier onset of action than antidepressant drugs. It has been found to be effective in the treatment of a number of psychiatric and neurologic conditions, including mood disorders (particularly psychotic depression), psychosis and Parkinson's disease. It is particularly effective when there is abnormal motor activity, e.g. catatonia, stupor and parkinsonism. The main indications for the use of ECT include:

- depressive stupor;

- failure to eat or drink;

- high risk of suicide;

- depressive delusions;

- marked psychomotor retardation; and

- previous good response to ECT.

However, there remains a certain amount of apprehension from the general public and certain health professionals about the safety of ECT. In reality the most common side-effects are headache, dizziness and confusion on the day of treatment. The death rate is about 1 in 10 000, and there are no absolute contraindications to its use. There are known long-term memory problems after treatment with ECT, but these are associated with continuing depression or substance abuse[1]. Nevertheless, the exact mechanism of action of ECT remains unclear.

SLEEP DEPRIVATION

There is a wide body of literature to indicate that sleep deprivation can sometimes improve the mood of depressed patients[2]. Sleep deprivation can be used in several ways, including total sleep deprivation (TSD), partial sleep deprivation (PSD), phase-advance therapy and selective rapid eye movement sleep deprivation. TSD involves the patient staying awake for up to 40 h starting from the morning before the night of sleep deprivation. In PSD, patients may sleep for 4 h and are then asked to wake up at around 01:00 to 02:00 and remain awake the rest of the night and the following day. The phase-advance approach involves changing the sleep pattern without sleep deprivation, e.g. patients go to bed at 18:00 and get up at 01:00. The antidepressant effect of sleep deprivation is not clearly understood.

LIGHT THERAPY

Light treatment (phototherapy) is most closely associated with the treatment of seasonal affective disorder. There are a number of devices used in light therapy, the most researched being the light box, with white light and an illumination of 10 000 lux (see Figure 10.1). Patients using light boxes are usually recommended to sit within 1 m of the box (ensuring that they receive about 5000 lux) starting at 1.5 h/day. The evidence suggests that morning treatment is superior to evening treatment[3]. Depressive symptoms usually respond within 2–4 days, although relapse is common if treatment is discontinued. Light therapy has also shown some promising results for the treatment of other mood disorders (e.g. non-seasonal major depressive disorder, premenstrual dysphoric disorder and rapid cycling bipolar disorder)[2]. However, the evidence suggests that it is best used as an adjunct to antidepressant therapy in the treatment of non-seasonal major depression[4]. The action of light therapy appears to be mediated via the retina, although the mechanism of action of light is not understood. Side-effects include headaches, eyestrain, irritability and insomnia. Light-induced mania can occur in some individuals.

TRANSCRANIAL MAGNETIC STIMULATION

Transcranial magnetic stimulation (TMS) is currently being explored as a potential treatment for patients with psychiatric and neurologic disorders (e.g. depression and Parkinson's disease). Rapid TMS (rTMS) involves passing a rapidly alternating electrical current through a small coil attached to the scalp, thereby inducing an electromagnetic pulse, which induces a change in the ionic flow of surrounding brain tissue. Several studies have found that rTMS of the left dorsolateral prefrontal area in healthy volunteers produced a feeling of sadness, while stimulation of the right dorsolateral prefrontal area produced a feeling of happiness[5]. However, in depressed patients rTMS of the left dorsolateral pre-

frontal area produced significant improvement. The evidence for its efficacy is currently still rather limited, and further work is currently being carried out (see Figure 10.2).

REFERENCES

1. Freeman CP, Weeks D, Kendell RE. ECT: II: patients who complain. *Br J Psychiatry* 1980;137:17–25

2. Kasper S, Neumeister A. Non-pharmacological treatments for depression – focus on sleep deprivation and light therapy. In: Briley M, Montgomery SA, eds. *Antidepressant Therapy at the Dawn of the Third Millennium.* London: Martin Dunitz, 1998:255–78

3. Avery DH, Khan A, Dager SR, Cox GB, Dunner DL. Bright light treatment of winter depression: morning versus evening light. *Acta Psychiatr Scand* 1990;82:335–8

4. Neuhaus IM, Rosenthal NE. Light therapy as a treatment modality for affective disorders. In: Honig A, Van Praag HH, eds. *Depression: neurobiological, psychopathological and therapeutic advances.* Chichester, John Wiley, 1997

5. Puri BK, Lewis SW. Transcranial magnetic stimulation in psychiatric research. *Br J Psychiatry* 1996;169:675–7

Psychologic therapies

COGNITIVE–BEHAVIOR THERAPY

Cognitive–behavior therapy (CBT)[1] is one of the most extensively researched and widely adopted psychological treatments for depression. It is based on the assumption that depressive moods are perpetuated and maintained through irrational beliefs and a distorted attitude toward the self, the environment and the future. In essence depression is argued to result from cognitions and not mood and postulates that there are three maladaptive elements of depression:

- a cognitive triad of recurrent negative views that directly shape how the person:

    - sees themselves (negative self-concept, e.g. worthless);

    - the world (overestimation of demands, e.g. life is meaningless); and

    - the future (e.g. hopeless).

- irrational schemata based on the past and logical errors that pervade the assessment of oneself and life events; and

- a number of typical processing errors, through which perceptions of events are distorted.

Examples of processing errors include:

- selective abstraction (attending only to negative aspects of experience);

- arbitrary inference (jumping to conclusions on inadequate evidence); and

- over-generalization (making judgements on the basis of single events).

During CBT, patients are helped to identify their maladaptive assumptions and processing errors, and then challenge them by monitoring their experience and associated emotional states. CBT sessions are standardized and last between 15 and 20 min. As 'homework' patients are asked to perform certain tasks, such as keeping a daily record of activities and listing negative thoughts as they occur. This is often complemented by behavioral techniques, such as scheduling pleasurable tasks and breaking seemingly insurmountable problems into smaller, achievable parts (Table 1).

Cognitive therapy is particularly effective when combined with antidepressant therapy, and has been found effective in preventing relapse when given in monthly 'booster sessions' after successful acute treatment with antidepressant drugs[2].

PROBLEM-SOLVING TREATMENT

Problem-solving treatment is a relatively new psychological intervention for depression. It is a brief and practical psychologic intervention that has been found to be effective in the treatment of depressive disorders in primary care[3,4]. Depressive disorders are known to be linked with stressful life events, and depressed patients may be less able to cope with these stresses in a clear

Table 1 Techniques used in cognitive–behavior therapy for depression

Keeping a daily record of activities and negative thoughts
Monitoring negative thoughts associated with worsening of mood
Challenging negative thoughts
Using imagination to 'replay' events
Questioning the assumptions that lead to negative thoughts
Planning rewarding activities throughout the day
Praising oneself for achievements
Dividing complex tasks into achievable components
Anticipating performance in challenging situations

problem-focussed way. The rationale for problem-solving treatment is that symptoms are caused by everyday problems, which can be resolved by the technique of problem-solving, and that resolution of problems leads to reduction in symptoms.

Two studies have evaluated the effectiveness of problem-solving treatment for major depression in primary care settings in the United Kingdom[3,4]. In these studies, problem-solving treatment was delivered in six sessions over 12 weeks as an acute treatment for depression. The first study found problem-solving to be similarly effective to amitriptyline, in patients with major depression. There were also fewer patient dropouts with problem-solving treatment (7%) than with amitriptyline (19%). All patients receiving the problem-solving approach found it either helpful or very helpful[5]. The second study assessed whether the combination of problem-solving treatment and antidepressant drugs (a selective serotonin reuptake inhibitor antidepressant) was more effective than either treatment given alone, in patients with major depression. It also compared delivery of the problem-solving technique by practice nurses and general practitioners. Problem-solving treatment was equally effective when provided alone or in combination with antidepressant therapy and when provided by nurses or general practitioners.

At present it is unknown whether problem-solving treatment is effective in the long-term treatment of depression, through reducing the rate of relapses or recurrence of illness. Depression in primary care usually occurs in the context of psychosocial problems[5], which may persist even if depressive symptoms resolve. As problem-solving treatment teaches patients a technique to enable them to resolve problems in a structured and logical way, it may protect patients against future relapse. However, it is uncertain whether problem-solving treatment is effective in older patients, or whether it is effective in patients with depressive disorders other than major depression.

NON-DIRECTIVE COUNSELING

In non-directive counseling the counselor takes a predominantly passive rather than an advisory role, and generally restricts their interventions to comments about the emotional content of their client's sessions.

One such form of counseling is the 'client-centered' approach developed by Carl Rogers in the 1940s and 1950s, the essence of which is to provide an atmosphere conducive to client growth and 'self-actualization'.

In a recent randomized controlled trial comparing non-directive counseling, CBT and 'usual' general practitioner care for patients with depression, it was found that in the short term (4 months) either psychologic therapy was a more effective treatment for depression than usual general practitioner care[6,7]. There was no significant difference between the psychologic therapies and, in addition, both were significantly more cost effective than usual care in the short term. However, at 12 months there was no difference between the three treatment groups in terms of outcome or cost-effectiveness.

INTERPERSONAL THERAPY

Interpersonal therapy (IPT) developed from the 'neo-Freudian' ideas of Harry Stack Sullivan (1892–1949). The basic assumptions of IPT are that emotional problems are a result of problematic interpersonal relationships experienced during childhood: primarily those between child and parents, but also between siblings and significant others. The consequences of problematic interpersonal relationships were argued to be maladaptive ways of dealing with life.

IPT was developed as a structured psychological treatment for problems in relation to the personal roles and interpersonal relationships of depressed patients. IPT defines four main interpersonal areas that are commonly associated with major depression: (1) abnormal grief reaction; (2) interpersonal role disputes; (3) difficult role transitions (e.g. developmental landmarks, career changes); and (4) interpersonal deficits (e.g. inadequate social skills). Therapy sessions are designed to be standardized and brief (15–20 min). Clear goals are set and progress monitored, and new coping strategies are tried out by the patient as 'homework strategies'.

IPT can be a useful treatment of the acute, continuation and maintenance phases of depression. Trials have shown IPT may be as effective as imipramine in acute treatment of depression[8]. However, there is some evidence that patients may require good social functioning as a pre-requisite to take full advantage of the interpersonal strategies to recover from depression.

BEREAVEMENT COUNSELING

Parkes[9] reviewed several studies assessing the efficacy of bereavement counseling. His findings suggested that professional services and professionally supported volunteer and self-help services were capable of reducing the risk of psychiatric and psychosomatic disorders resulting from bereavement. In addition Parkes later evaluated the efficacy of a hospice bereavement service[10]. A significant association was found between 'high-risk' and 'poor-outcome' in those who were unsupported. Bereavement support reduced the risk in 'high-risk' groups to about that of low-risk groups. Support also reduced the consumption of drugs, alcohol and tobacco by the bereaved and reduced the number of symptoms attributable to anxiety and tension. In general, bereavement services are best targeted at those who are at high risk and unsupported (or perceive their families as unsupportive).

There are a number of risk factors associated with poor outcome in bereavement, including:

- sudden or unexpected death;

- miscarriage or death of a baby, child or sibling;

- multiple prior bereavements;

- a history of mental illness (e.g. depression, anxiety);

- cohabiting partner, same-sex partner, extra-marital relationship (may result in 'disenfranchised' grief);

- ambivalent or dependent relationship with the person who has been lost;

- death with a potential stigma (e.g. AIDS, suicide);

- deaths resulting from accidents where bereaved may be responsible;

- deaths from murder or involving legal proceedings; and

- where a postmortem and inquest is required.

REFERENCES

1. Beck AT, Rush AJ, Shaw BF, Emery G. *Cognitive Therapy of Depression*. New York: Guilford Press, 1970

2. Fava GA, Rafanelli C, Grandi S, *et al*. Six-year outcome for cognitive behavioral treatment of residual symptoms in major depression. *Am J Psychiatry* 1998;155:1443–5

3. Mynors-Wallis LM, Gath DH, Lloyd-Thomas AR, *et al*. Randomised controlled trial comparing problem-solving treatment with amitriptyline and placebo for major depression in primary care. *Br Med J* 1995;310:441–5

4. Mynors-Wallis LM, Gath DH, Day A, *et al*. Randomised controlled trial of problem-solving treatment, antidepressant medication and combined treatment for major depression in primary care. *Br Med J* 2000:320;26–30

5. Sireling LI, Freeling P, Paykel ES, *et al*. Depression in general practice: clinical features and comparison with out-patients. *Br J Psychiatry* 1985;147:119–26

6. Ward E, King M, Lloyd M, *et al*. Randomised controlled trial of non-directive counselling, cognitive–behaviour therapy, and usual general practitioner care for patients with depression. I: Clinical effectiveness. *Br Med J* 2000;321:1383–8

7. Bower P, Byford S, Sibbald B, *et al*. Randomised controlled trial of non-directive counselling, cognitive–behaviour therapy, and usual general practitioner care for patients with depression. II: Cost effectiveness. *Br Med J* 2000;321:1389–92

8. DiMascio A, Weissman M, Prusoff B, Neu C, Zwilling M, Klerman G. Differential symptom reduction by drugs and psychotherapy in acute depression. *Arch Gen Psychiatry* 1979;36:1450–6

9. Parkes CM. Bereavement counselling: does it work? *Br Med J* 1980;281:3–6

10. Parkes CM. Evaluation of a bereavement service. *J Preventative Psychiatry* 1981;1:179–88

CHAPTER 12

Sexual problems and depression

INTRODUCTION

Community-based studies suggest that sexual problems are relatively common. Dunn and colleagues[1] carried out an anonymous postal survey of a random sample of 4000 adult patients registered at four general practices in the UK. A total of 789 men and 979 women completed the questionnaire, which equated to a response rate of 44% with a median age of 50 years. Current sexual problems were reported by 34% of men and 41% of women. The most common are shown in Table 1.

Sexual problems are common in patients with depression. Many patients with depression experience a reduction in sexual interest and satisfaction, which is often associated with other 'biological' symptoms of depression, including weight loss, reduction in sleep and loss of energy. Araujo and coworkers[2] compared the sexual function of men (aged 40–70 years) with depression with non-depressed age- and sex-matched controls, and found that 35% of depressed compared to 0% of non-depressed control men experienced erectile dysfunction. Premature or delayed ejaculation was described by 38% and 47% of depressed men, compared to 0% and 6% of the non-depressed controls, respectively.

NEUROTRANSMITTERS AND SEXUAL FUNCTION

Many neurotransmitters are involved in normal sexual function and their actions are complex and interconnected. They include dopamine, serotonin (5-hydroxy-tryptamine – 5-HT), norepinephrine, acetylcholine, γ-aminobutyric acid (GABA), oxytocin, nitric oxide, arg-vasopressin, angiotensin II, gonadotropin-releasing hormone, substance P, neuropeptide Y and cholecystokinin-8. Four neurotransmitters are of particular interest in relation to depression: dopamine, serotonin, norepinephrine and acetylcholine.

Dopamine facilitates sexual activity, probably through actions within the central nervous system. An increase in central dopamine, for example through the administration of dopamine agonists such as levodopa and bromocriptine (used in the treatment of Parkinson's disease), may increase sexual activity in both humans and animals. In clinical practice dopamine antagonists, such as conventional antipsychotic drugs, are often linked to the development of sexual dysfunction.

The role of serotonin in sexual behavior is not understood fully. Increased transmission within central serotonergic pathways produces a reduction in sexual arousal, while increased transmission in the peripheral pathways produces a reduction in penile sensation and ejaculation. These inhibitory effects are believed to be mediated by 5-HT_2 receptors. These findings correspond with the clinical observation that sexual dysfunction associated with serotonin re-uptake inhibitors can be reversed by 5-HT_2 antagonists. Serotonergic pathways also interconnect with noradrenergic and dopaminergic pathways.

Norepinephrine plays a significant role in sexual behavior, with both central and peripheral actions. Increased peripheral action can impair sexual performance by promoting detumescence and impotence. Priapism is a side-effect sometimes seen with drugs with high α_1-adrenergic blocking potential combined with minimum anticholinergic effects (e.g. trazodone or

Table 1 Common sexual problems associated with depression

Men	Women
Erectile dysfunction (22%)	Vaginal dryness (19%)
Premature ejaculation (11%)	Infrequent orgasm (17%).

thioridazine). Finally, acetylcholine may reduce arousal and the threshold for ejaculation in men. In addition, optimal sexual function probably depends on a balance of adrenergic and cholinergic effects.

ANTIDEPRESSANT DRUGS AND SEXUAL FUNCTION

Antidepressant drugs are sometimes associated with the development of sexual dysfunction. The incidence of antidepressant-induced sexual problems is probably underestimated, owing to a combination of under-reporting by patients and general lack of discussion about sexual problems between doctors and patients. Most antidepressant drugs have been found to cause sexual problems in at least some patients.

Of particular interest has been the reports that a significant number of those taking selective serotonin reuptake inhibitors (SSRIs) experience sexual dysfunction[3]. SSRIs are associated with the development of most forms of sexual problems, particularly delayed ejaculation in men and anorgasmia in women (see Table 2). Table 3 shows a number of pharmacologic approaches to the treatment of sexual dysfunction.

Table 2 Sexual dysfunction with selective serotonin reuptake inhibitors[4]

	Fluoxetine (n=129)	Fluvoxamine (n=29)	Paroxetine (n=59)	Sertraline (n=46)
Mean dosage (mg)	20.9	114	20.6	88.4
Decreased libido	46.5	34.5	50.8	45.7
Delayed ejaculation/orgasm	47.3	44.8	54.2	54.7
Anorgasmia	34.1	6.9	32.2	13.1
Total sexual dysfunction	51.9	48.3	54.2	56.5

Table 3 Pharmacologic approaches to treating sexual dysfunction

Continue with the same treatment.	Some treatment-emergent sexual dysfunction may remit with time.
Delayed dosing	Some patients find improvement by delaying their medication until after sexual activity. This may be helpful with antidepressants that have a short half-life, e.g. paroxetine.
Drug holidays	Treatment is interrupted briefly, for 1–2 days, before sexual activity. This method appears to be beneficial with antidepressants with a short half-life but not those with a longer half-life, e.g. fluoxetine. However, the 'planning' of sexual activity required in this approach may be unacceptable for some.
Reduction in drug dose	Sexual dysfunction may be more common with higher doses of medication. For some, a dose reduction may be effective at reducing sexual problems. However, clinicians must be cautious, as this may also reduce the therapeutic value of the medication in the treatment of the patient's depression and increase the risk of relapse.
Withdrawal of medication	If the sexual problems are particularly distressing to the patient then withdrawal of medication may be considered. Recovery may vary according to the half-life of the medication. However, as with dose reduction there is the risk of relapse.
Treatment substitution	Some patients may benefit from switching from one drug to another. For example, Koutouvidis and colleagues found switching patients with SSRI-induced sexual dysfunction from their current medication to mirtazapine was successful in resolving sexual problems[5].

Adjunctive treatment	Class	Example
A number of adjunctive compounds have been used to treat drug-induced sexual problems. The cholinergic agonists neostigmine and bethanechol have been reported to reverse anorgasmia linked with tricyclic antidepressants. Dopamine agonists such as amantadine have also been found to be helpful in anorgasmia associated with some antidepressants. The 5-HT$_{1A}$ partial agonist buspirone has also been used in the management of SSRI-emergent sexual problems. Unfortunately, there have been few double-blind placebo controlled trials of these adjunctive treatments in patients with depression. Newer drug treatments, e.g. sildenafil, may prove to be better at treating some treatment-emergent sexual problems.	serotonin antagonist	cyproheptadine, mianserin
	5-HT$_{1A}$ partial agonist	buspirone
	adrenergic antagonist	yohimbine, fluparoxan
	cholinergic agonist	neostigmine, bethanechol
	dopamine agonists	amantadine, dextroamphetamine, pemoline
	newer drug treatments	sildenafil
	complementary approaches	Ginkgo biloba

REFERENCES

1. Dunn KM, Croft PR, Hackett GI. Sexual problems: a study of the prevalence and need for health care in the general population. *Fam Pract* 1998;15:519–24

2. Araujo AB, Durante R, Feldman HA, Goldstein I, McKinlay JB. The relationship between depressive symptoms and male erectile dysfunction: cross-sectional results from the Massachusetts Male Aging Study. *Psychosom Med* 1998;60:458–65

3. Baldwin DS. Depression and sexual dysfunction. *Br Med Bull* 2001;57:81–99

4. Montejo AI, Llorca G, Izquierdo JA, *et al.* Sexual dysfunction secondary to SSRIs. A comparative analysis in 308 patients [in Spanish]. *Actas Luso Esp Neurol Psiquiatr Cienc Afines* 1996;24:311–21

5. Koutouvidis N, Pratikakis M, Fotiadou A. The use of mirtazepine in a group of 11 patients following poor compliance to selective serotonin reuptake inhibitor treatment due to sexual dysfunction. *Int Clin Psychopharmacol* 1999;14:253–5

BIBLIOGRAPHY

Segraves RT. Effects of psychotropic drugs on human erection and ejaculation. *Arch Gen Psychiatry* 1989;46:275–84

Wilson CA. Pharmacological targets for the control of male and female sexual behaviour. In: Riley A, Peet M, Wilson C, eds, *Sexual Pharmacology*. Oxford, UK: Oxford Medical Publications, 1993:1-58

Section II   Depression Illustrated

List of illustrations

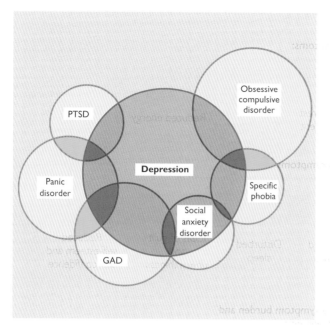

Figure 1.1 The comorbidity of depression and anxiety

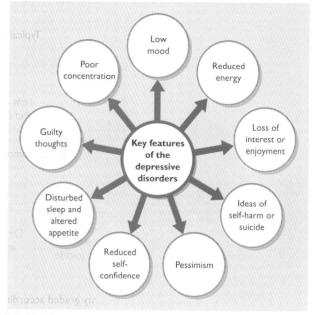

Figure 1.2 Key features of the depressive disorders

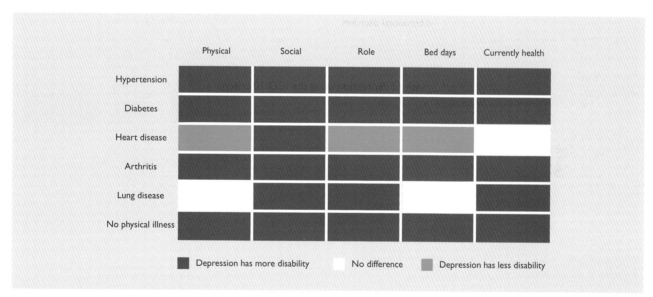

Figure 1.3 Disability in medical conditions. Functioning in 11 242 patients in Medical Outcomes Study. Adapted with permission from Wells KB, Stewart A, Hays RD, et al. The functioning and well-being of depressed patients. Results from the Medical Outcomes Study. *JAMA* 1989;262:914–19

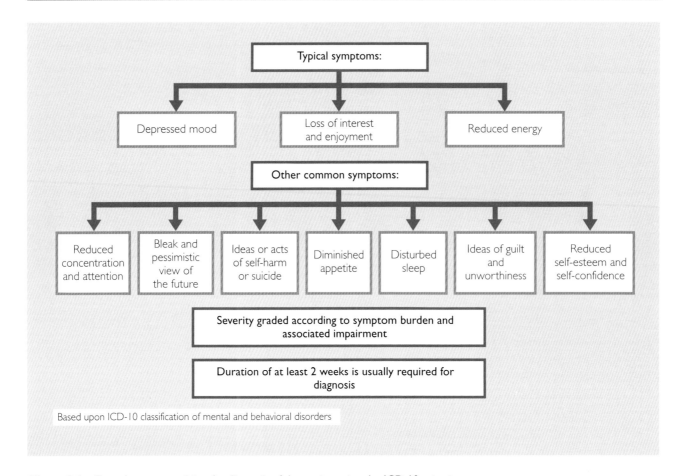

Figure 2.1   Flow chart summarizing the diagnosis of depression using the ICD-10 criteria

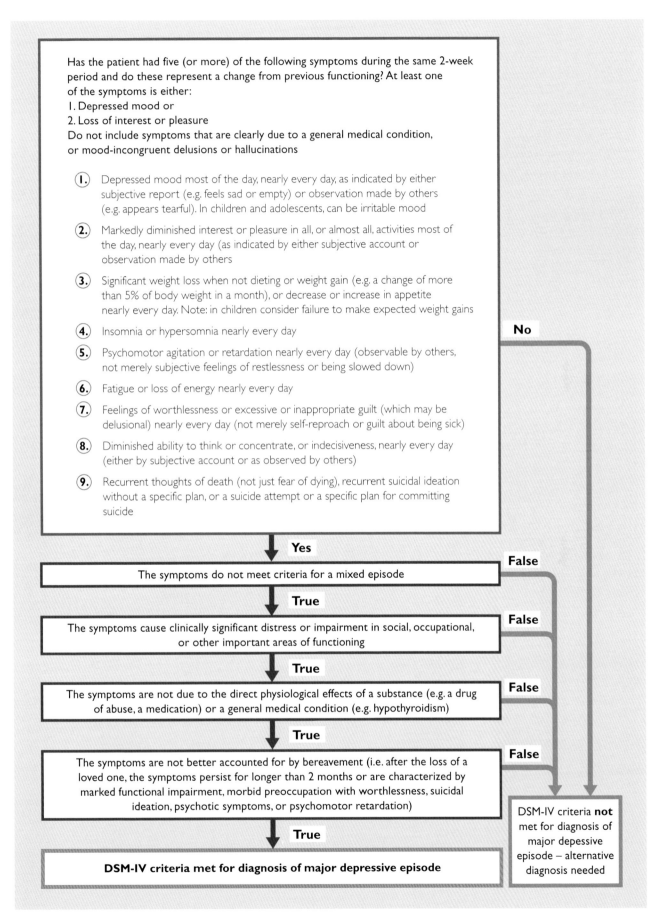

Figure 2.2 Flow chart summarizing the diagnosis of major depressive episodes using the DSM-IV criteria

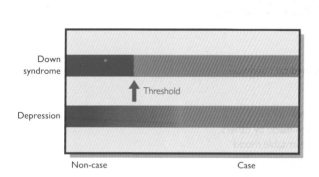

Figure 2.3 Graph comparing the 'caseness' of depression versus a more 'definite' diagnosis

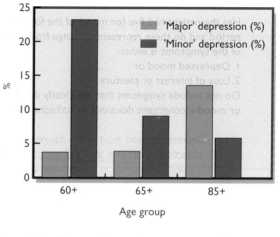

Figure 2.4 The incidence of depression in old age. As can be seen, the proportion of 'major' to 'minor' increases with age. Data from Katona CLE. *The Epidemiology of Old Age*. Chichester, UK: Wiley, 1994:33

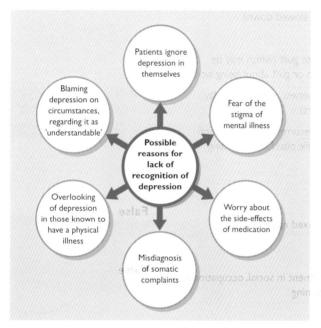

Figure 3.1 Reasons for the lack of recognition of depression

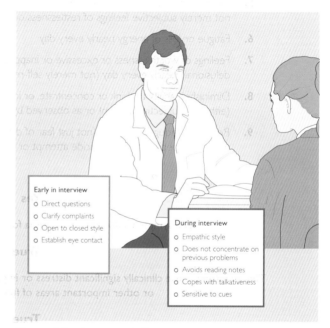

Figure 3.2 Interview skills

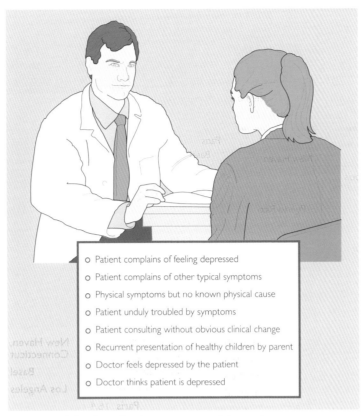

Figure 3.3 Cues for the recognition of depression

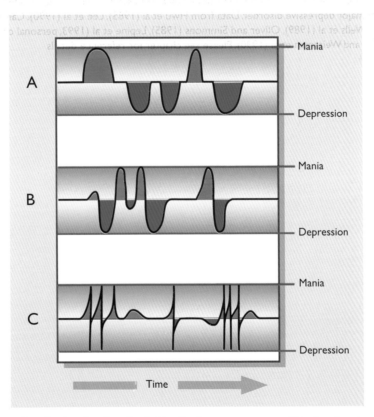

Figure 4.1 Patterns of illness found in bipolar disorder. A, Usually the two extremes of bipolar disorder occur in separate episodes with a period of recovery between episodes. B, Some individuals may suffer more dramatic mood swings from depression to mania within the course of a single episode. C, Occasionally mixed states are observed where the mania and depressive illness occur at the same time

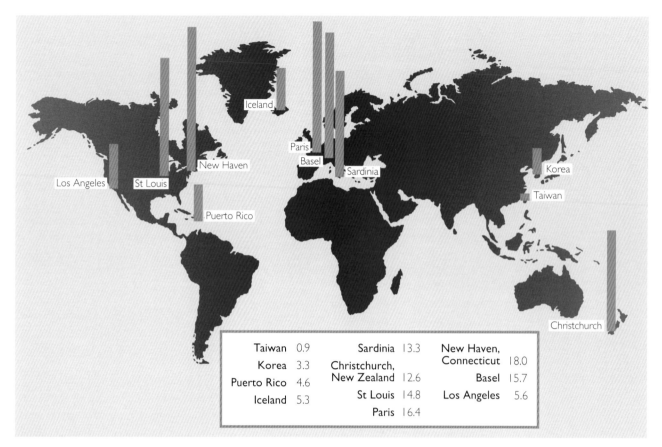

Figure 4.2   Recent rates of major depression in both men and women from selected countries worldwide. Figures represent the lifetime prevalence rates (%) of major depressive disorder. Data from Hwu et al (1985), Lee et al (1990), Canino et al (1987), Stefansson et al (1991), Carta et al (1995), Wells et al (1989), Oliver and Simmons (1985), Lepine et al (1993, personal communication), Weissman and Myers (1978), Wacker (1985) and Weissman et al (1990). Please see chapter for reference details

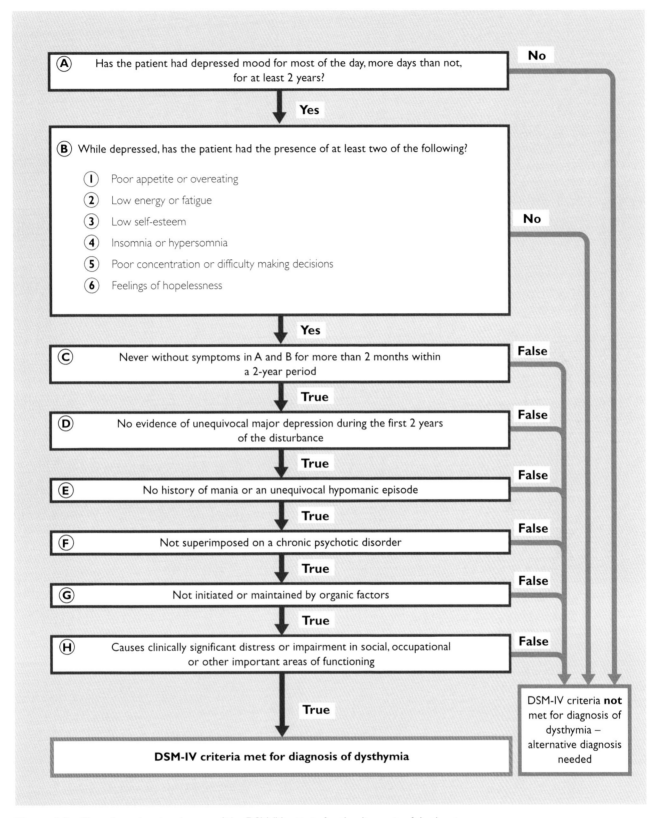

Figure 4.3   Flow chart showing the use of the DSM-IV criteria for the diagnosis of dysthymia

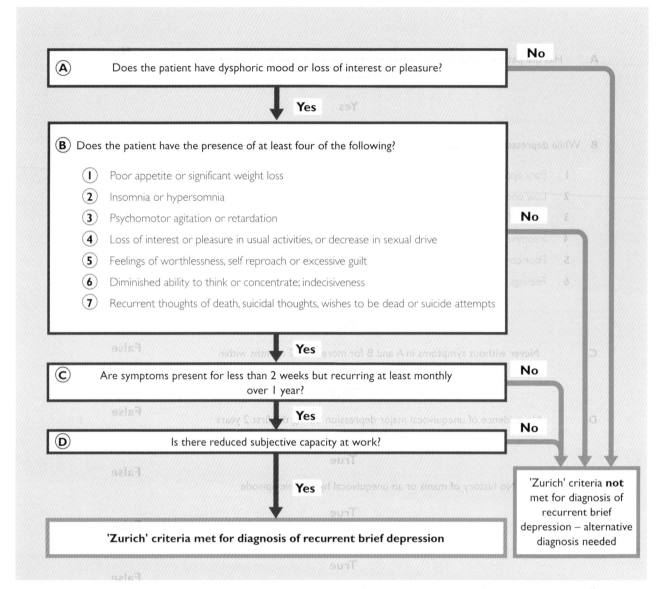

Figure 4.4   Flow chart describing the use of the 'Zurich' criteria for the diagnosis of recurrent brief depression

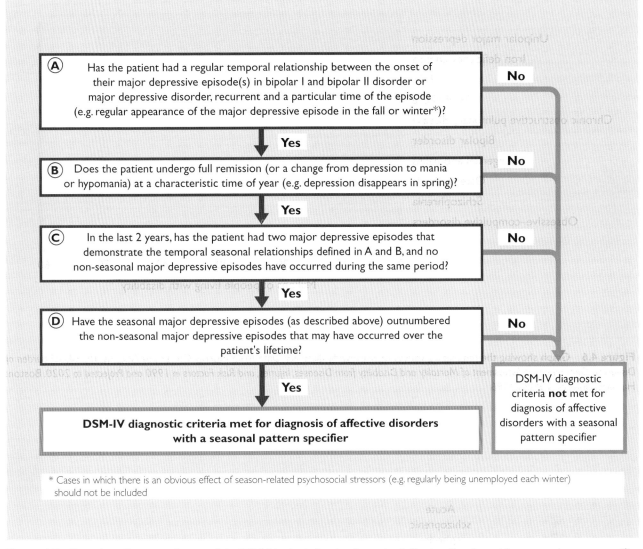

(A) Has the patient had a regular temporal relationship between the onset of their major depressive episode(s) in bipolar I and bipolar II disorder or major depressive disorder, recurrent and a particular time of the episode (e.g. regular appearance of the major depressive episode in the fall or winter*)?   **No**

Yes

(B) Does the patient undergo full remission (or a change from depression to mania or hypomania) at a characteristic time of year (e.g. depression disappears in spring)?   **No**

Yes

(C) In the last 2 years, has the patient had two major depressive episodes that demonstrate the temporal seasonal relationships defined in A and B, and no non-seasonal major depressive episodes have occurred during the same period?   **No**

Yes

(D) Have the seasonal major depressive episodes (as described above) outnumbered the non-seasonal major depressive episodes that may have occurred over the patient's lifetime?   **No**

Yes

DSM-IV diagnostic criteria met for diagnosis of affective disorders with a seasonal pattern specifier

DSM-IV diagnostic criteria **not** met for diagnosis of affective disorders with a seasonal pattern specifier

* Cases in which there is an obvious effect of season-related psychosocial stressors (e.g. regularly being unemployed each winter) should not be included

Figure 4.5   Flow chart illustrating the use of the DSM-IV criteria for the diagnosis of affective disorders with a seasonal pattern specifier

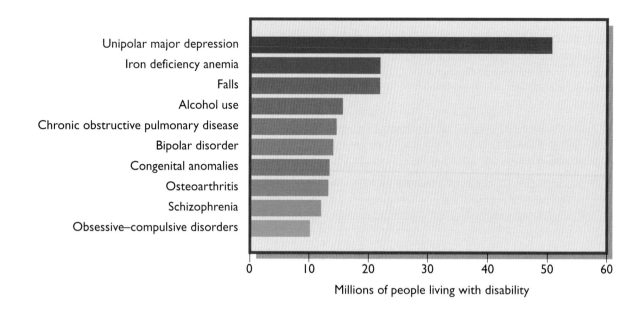

Figure 4.6   Graph showing the ten leading causes of worldwide disability. Data from Murray CJL, Lopez AD, eds. *The Global Burden of Disease: a Comprehensive Assessment of Mortality and Disability from Diseases, Injuries, and Risk Factors in 1990 and Projected to 2020.* Boston: Harvard University Press, 1996

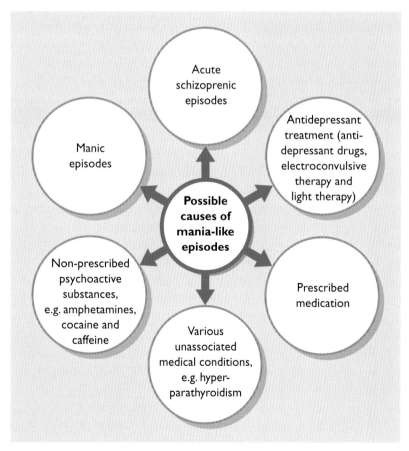

Figure 4.7   The causes of mania-like episodes

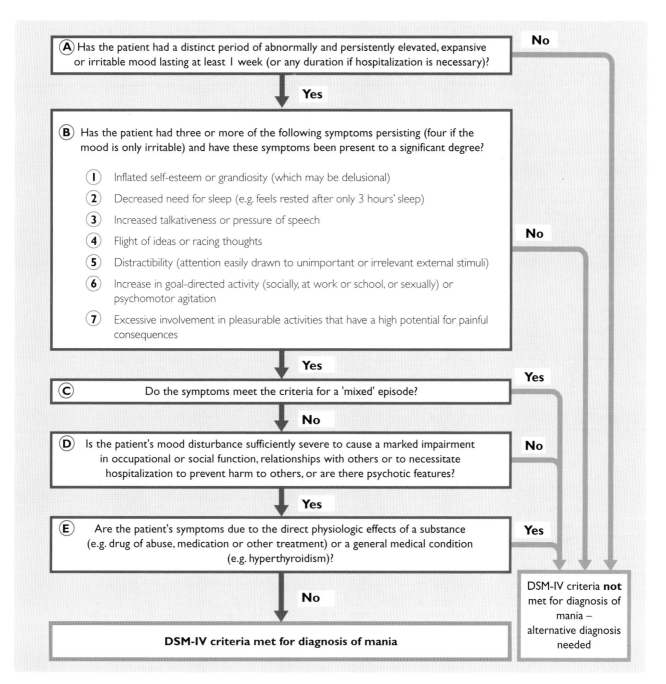

Figure 4.8   Flow chart illustrating the use of DSM-IV criteria for the diagnosis of mania

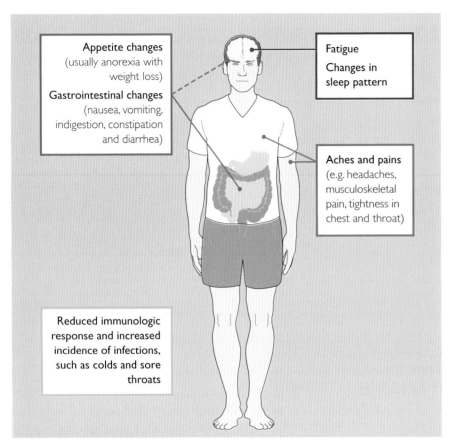

Figure 4.9   The physical symptoms of normal grief

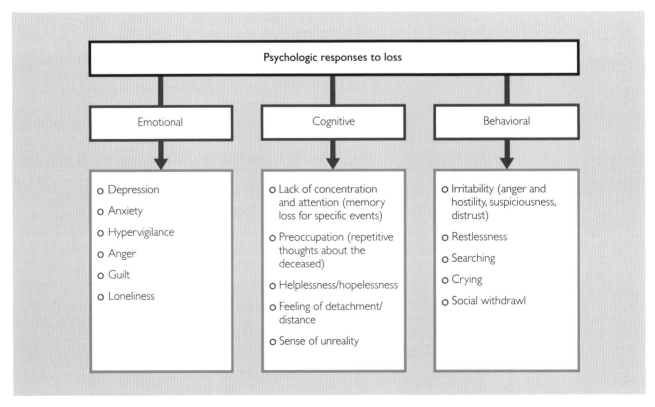

Figure 4.10   The psychologic responses to loss

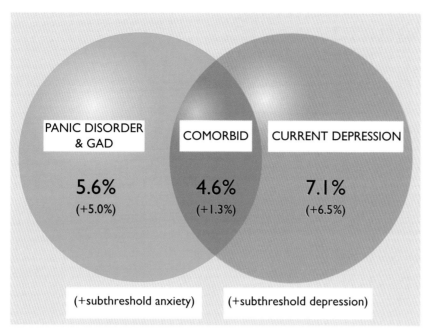

Figure 5.1 Comorbidity of ICD-10 anxiety and depressive disorders. Reproduced with permission from Sartorius N, Üstün TB, Lecrubier Y, Wittchen HU. Depression comorbid with anxiety: results from the WHO study on psychological disorders in primary health care. *Br J Psychiatry* 1996;suppl 30:38-43

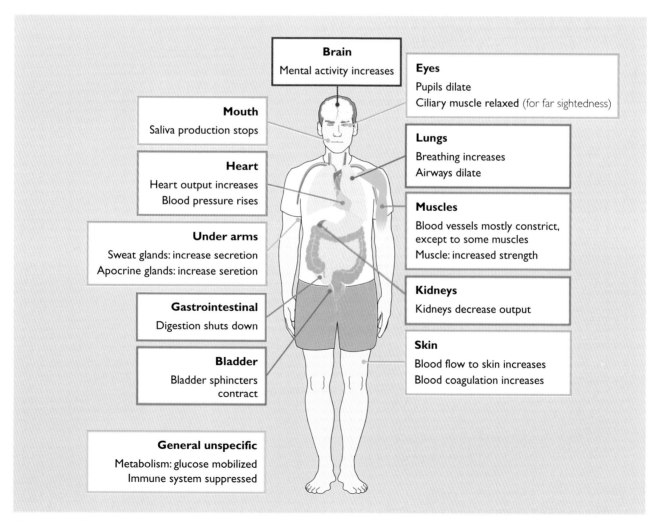

Figure 5.2 The physiologic response to 'flight or fight' stimuli

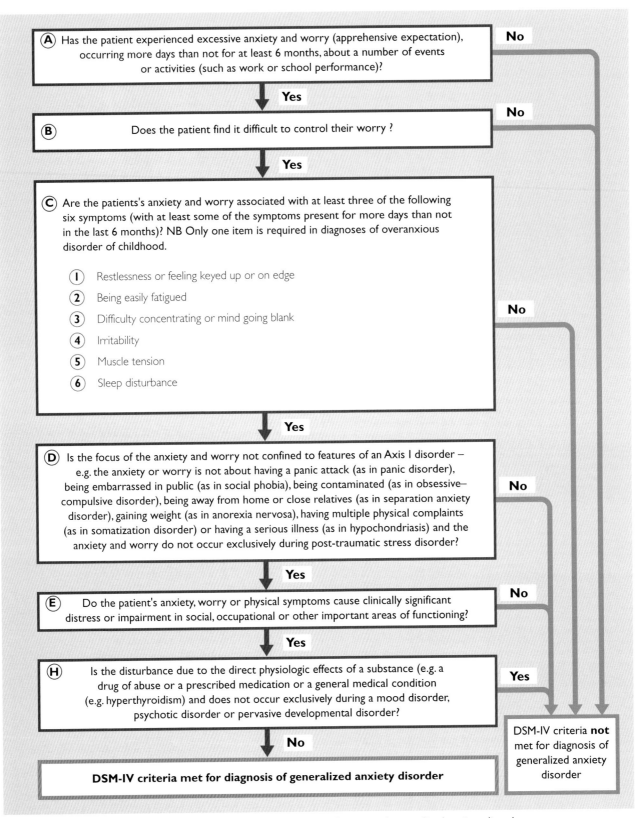

Figure 5.3 Flow chart describing the use of DSM-IV criteria for the diagnosis of generalized anxiety disorder

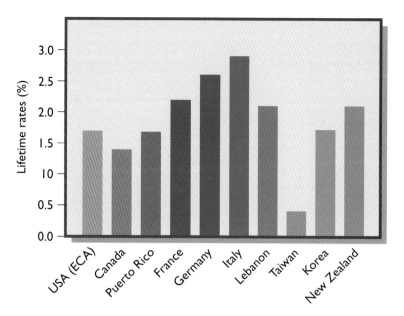

Figure 5.4 Lifetime rates of panic disorder. Data from Weissman MM, Bland RC, Canino GJ, *et al*. The cross-national epidemiology of panic disorder. *Arch Gen Psychiatry* 1997;54:305–9

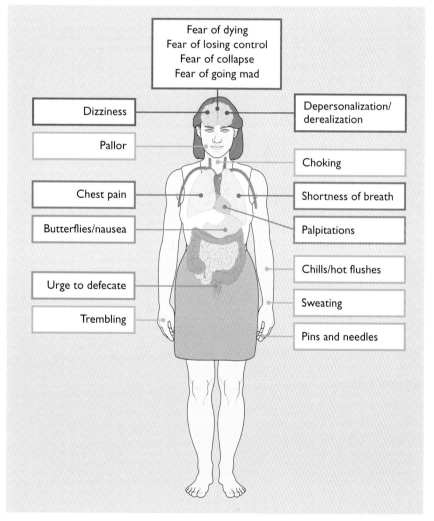

Figure 5.5 The symptoms of panic. Compare with Figure 5.2

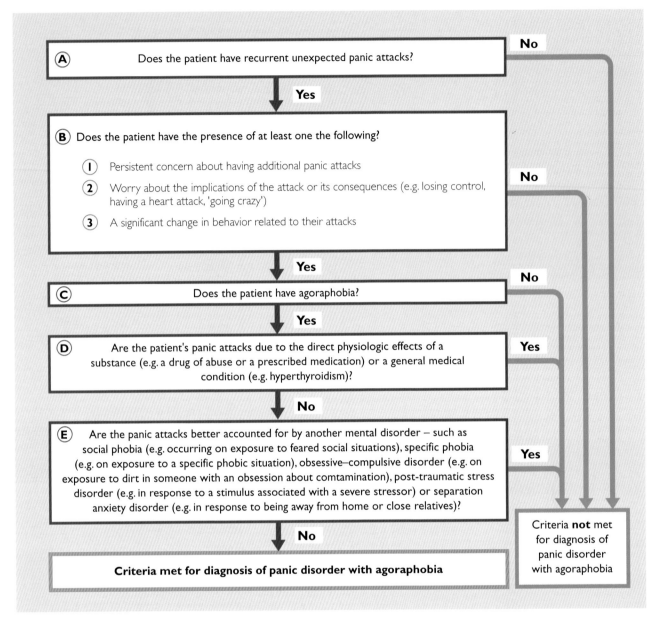

Figure 5.6 Flow chart describing the use of the DSM-IV criteria for the diagnosis of panic disorder with agoraphobia

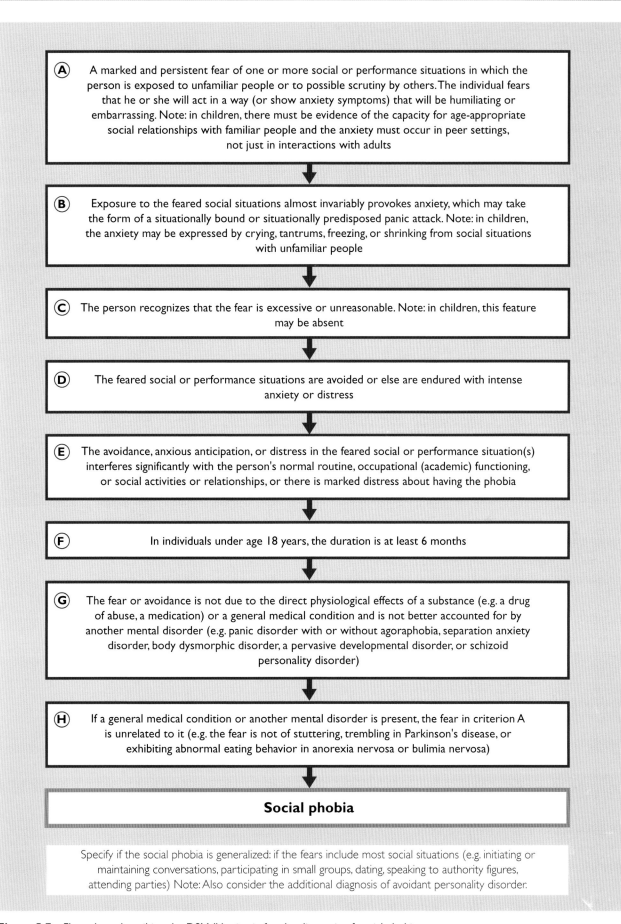

Figure 5.7　Flow chart describing the DSM-IV criteria for the diagnosis of social phobia

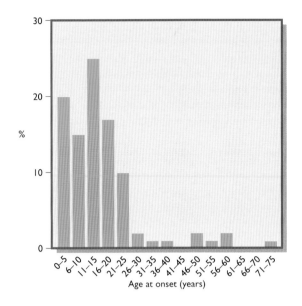

Figure 5.8 Age of onset of social phobia. Most cases of social phobia start before the age of 20 years. Reproduced and adapted with permission from Schneier FR, Johnson J, Hornig CD, Liebowitz MR, Weissman MM. Social phobia. Comorbidity and morbidity in an epidemiologic sample. *Arch Gen Psychiatry* 1992;49:282–8

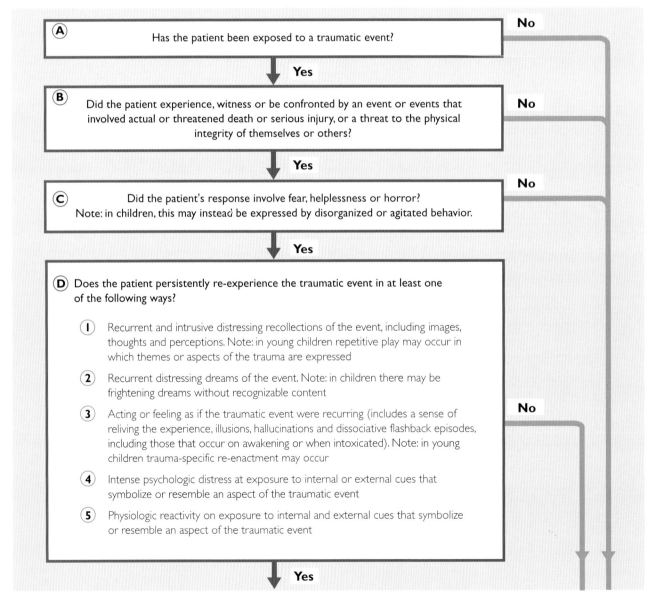

Figure 5.9 [Above and right] Flow chart illustrating the use of the DSM-IV criteria for the diagnosis of post-traumatic stress disorder

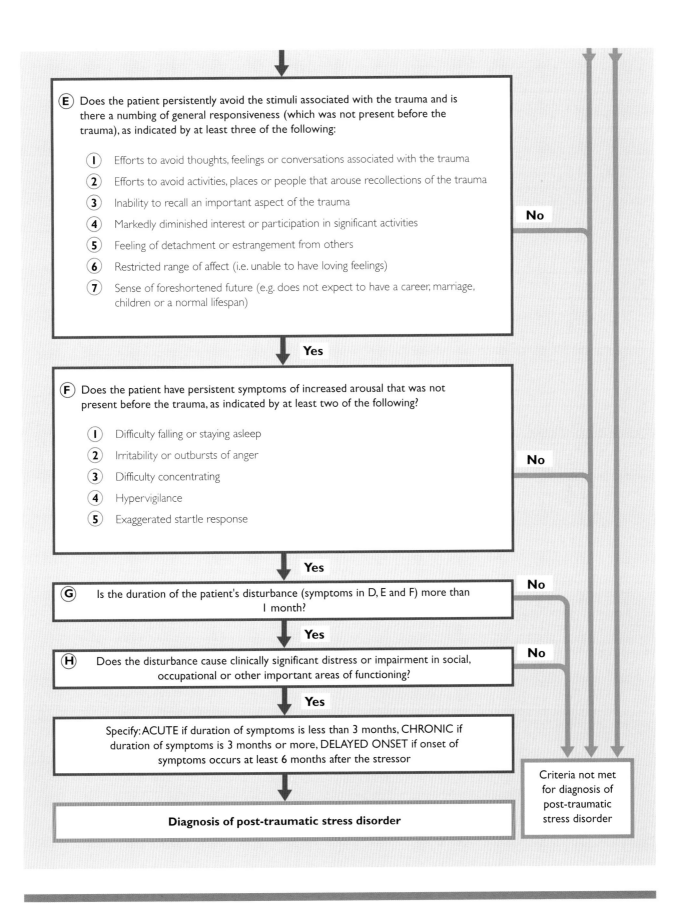

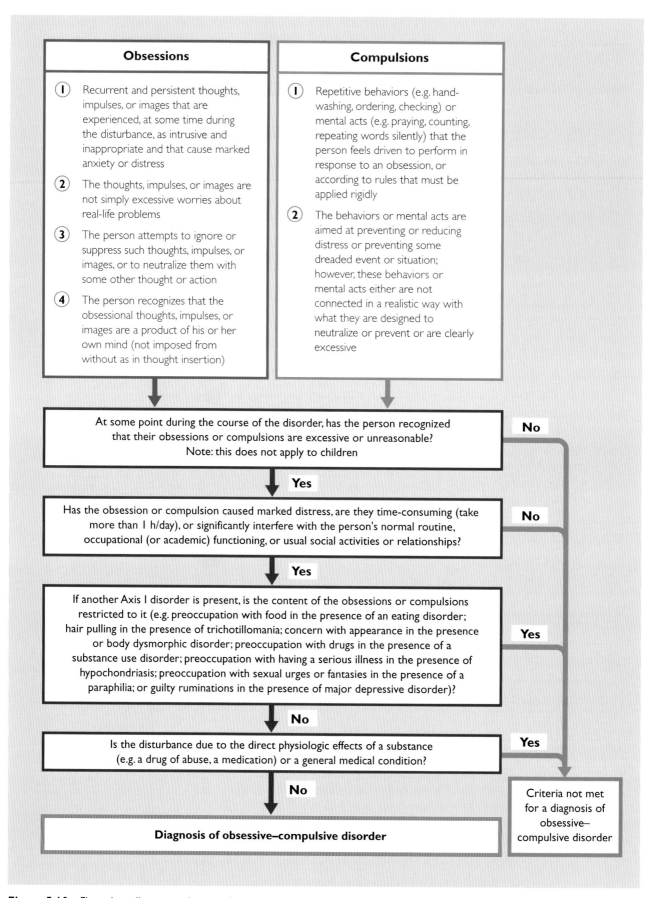

Figure 5.10 Flow chart illustrating the use of the DSM-IV criteria for the diagnosis of obsessive–compulsive disorder

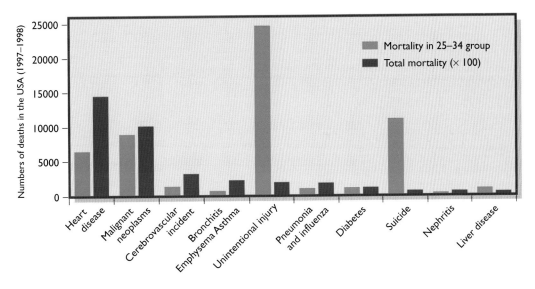

Figure 6.1 Comparative rates for cause of death in the USA. Data from the Center for Disease Control (http://webapp.cdc.gov/sasweb/ncipc/leadcaus.html)

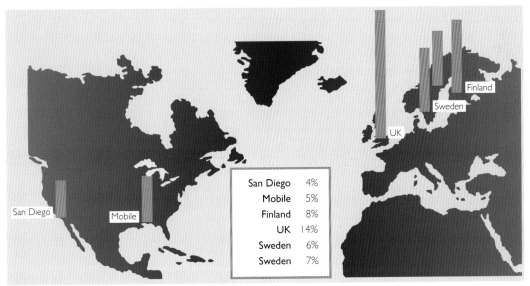

San Diego	4%
Mobile	5%
Finland	8%
UK	14%
Sweden	6%
Sweden	7%

Figure 6.2 Proportion of suicides due to antidepressant overdose in Europe and North America. Data from Isacsson (1994a), Rich (1997), Isometsa (1994), Jick (1995), Isacsson (1994b) and Isacsson (1997)

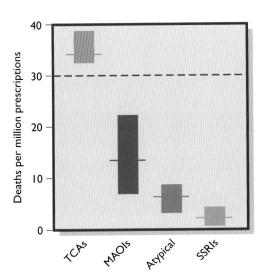

Figure 6.3 Comparison of overdose deaths per million prescriptions according to antidepressant class. Broken line represents the figure for all antidepressants. Data from Henry JA, Alexander CA, Sener EK. Relative mortality from overdose of antidepressants. *Br Med J* 1995;310:221–4

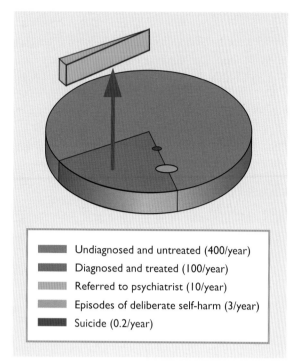

Figure 6.4 Prevalence of depression in general practice

Legend:
- Undiagnosed and untreated (400/year)
- Diagnosed and treated (100/year)
- Referred to psychiatrist (10/year)
- Episodes of deliberate self-harm (3/year)
- Suicide (0.2/year)

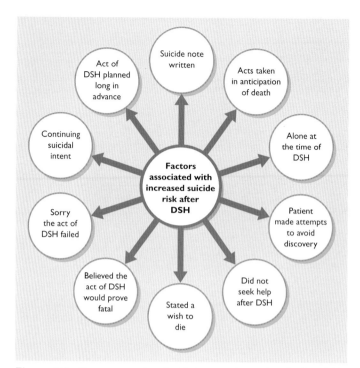

Figure 6.5 Factors associated with increased suicide risk after deliberate self-harm (DSH)

Factors associated with increased suicide risk after DSH:
- Act of DSH planned long in advance
- Suicide note written
- Acts taken in anticipation of death
- Alone at the time of DSH
- Patient made attempts to avoid discovery
- Did not seek help after DSH
- Stated a wish to die
- Believed the act of DSH would prove fatal
- Sorry the act of DSH failed
- Continuing suicidal intent

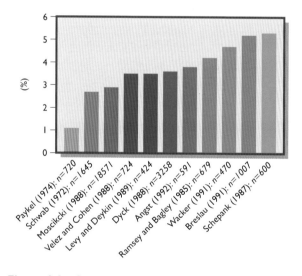

Figure 6.6 Community studies of the incidence of suicide attempts. Please see text for references

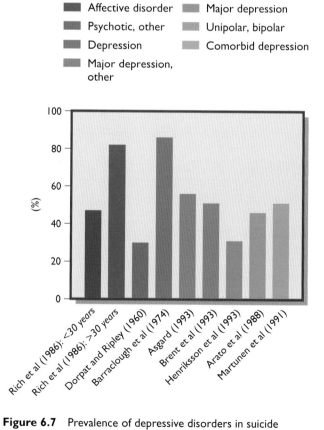

Legend:
- Affective disorder
- Affective disorder
- Psychotic, other
- Depression
- Major depression, other
- Major depression
- Major depression
- Unipolar, bipolar
- Comorbid depression

Figure 6.7 Prevalence of depressive disorders in suicide

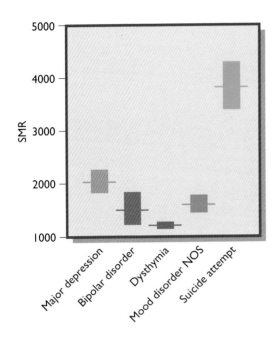

Figure 6.8 Suicide as an outcome of depression (standardized mortality ratio (SMR) (×100) ± confidence interval). Data from Harris EC, Barraclough B. Suicide as an outcome for mental disorders. A meta-analysis. *Br J Psychiatry* 1997;170:205–28

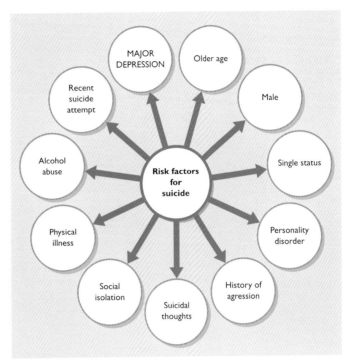

Figure 6.9 Risk factors for suicide

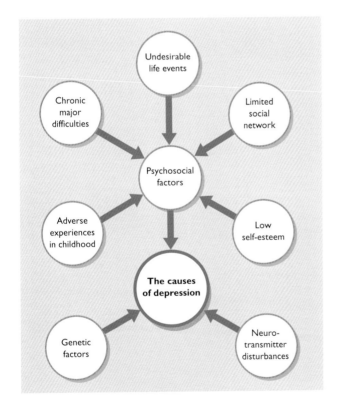

Figure 7.1 The etiology of depression

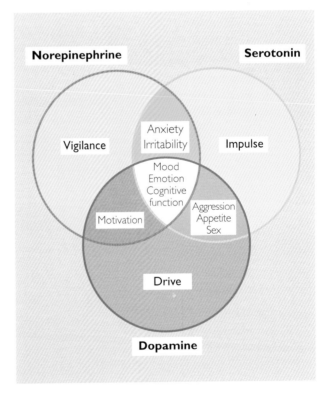

Figure 7.2 Neurotransmitters and their possible influence on psychopathology

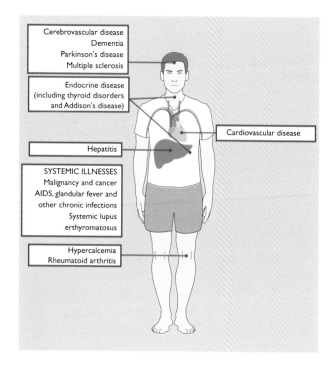

Figure 7.3 Examples of physical illness associated with depression

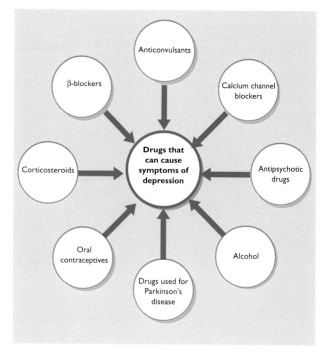

Figure 7.4 Drugs that can cause symptoms of depression

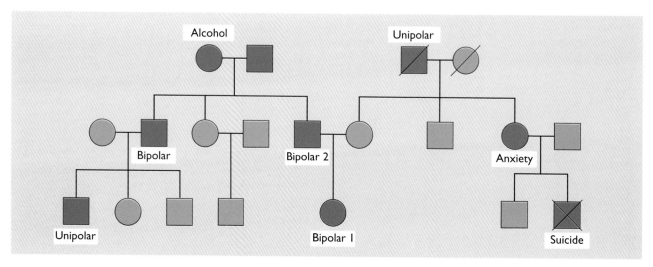

Figure 7.5 Genetic map of a typical family affected by the depressive disorders

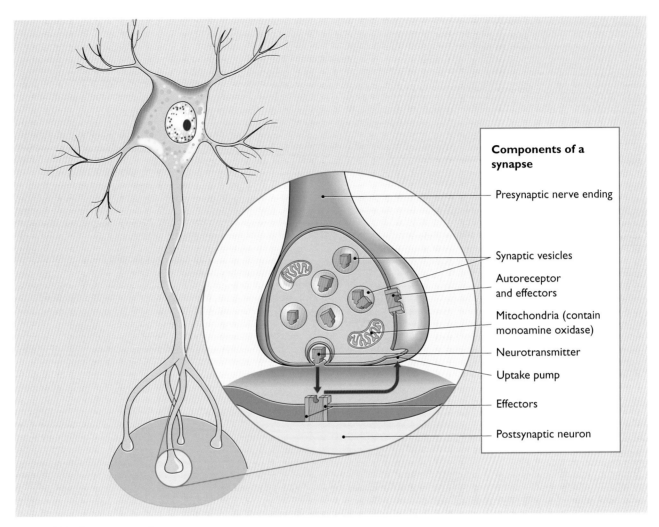

Figure 7.6 Components of a synapse

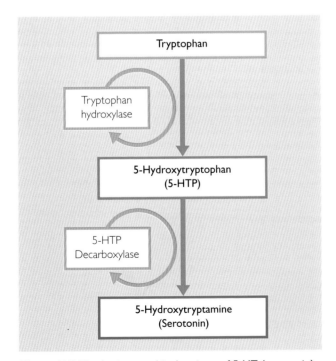

Figure 7.7 The basic neurobiochemistry of 5-HT (serotonin)

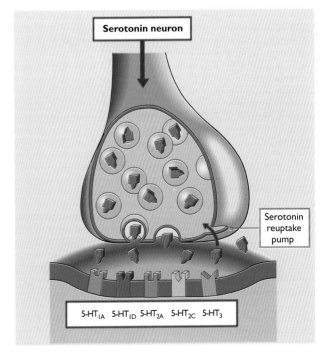

Figure 7.8 The 5-HT (serotonin) synapse

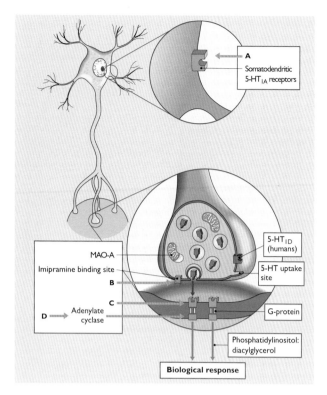

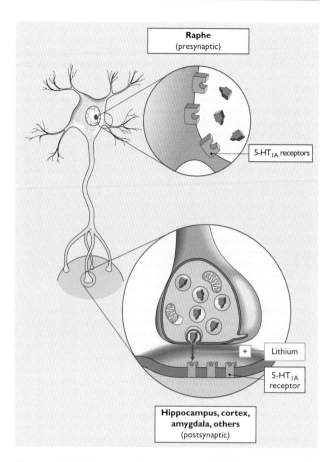

Figure 7.9 Possible neurobiochemical factors associated with depressed states. A, SSRIs and MAOIs desensitize the inhibitory 5-HT$_{1A}$ somatodendritic receptors; B, SSRIs and MAOIs desensitize the inhibitory autoreceptor on the presynaptic terminal. TCAs and SSRIs inhibit the reuptake of 5-HT into the nerve terminal after acute administration by binding to the serotonin transporter; C, Postsynaptic serotonin receptors activated by increased serotonin in the synaptic cleft; D, Information is translated from the receptor to the cell by second messenger systems

Figure 7.10 The neurobiochemistry of 5-HT$_{1A}$ receptors. 5-HT$_{1A}$ receptors may be somatodendritic or postsynaptic. Antidepressant drugs probably exert their action through effect at postsynatic 5-HT$_{1A}$ receptors

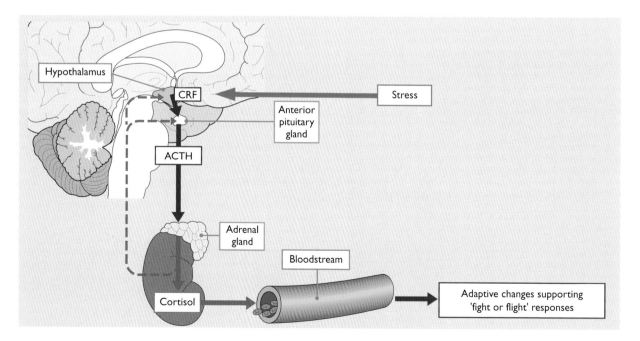

Figure 7.11 Adrenal gland function in terms of cortisol production. The hypothalamus–pituitary–adrenal axis may be disturbed in patients with chronic or resistant depression, with elevated cortisol levels and adrenal gland hypertrophy

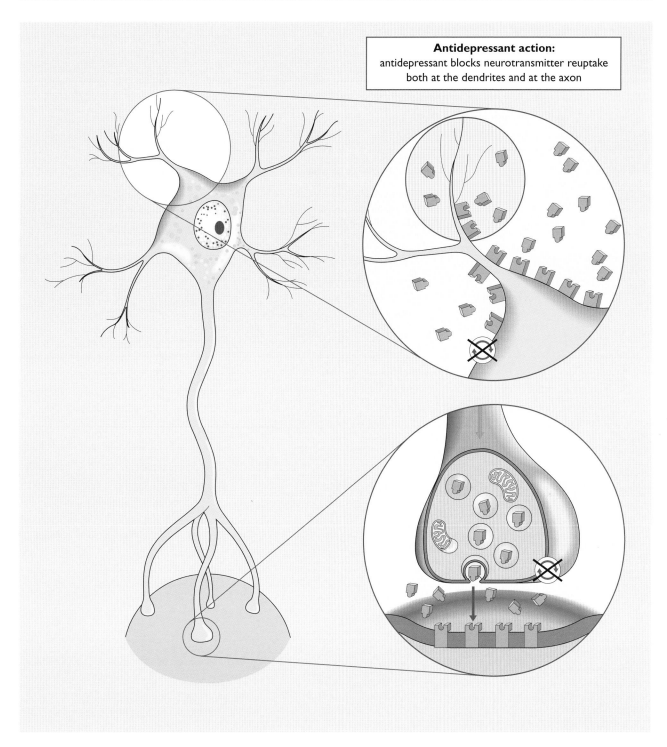

Figure 7.12 Downregulation of α_2 somatodendritic receptors by antidepressant drugs. Antagonism of α_2-autoreceptors increases the availability of norepinephrine at postsynaptic receptors

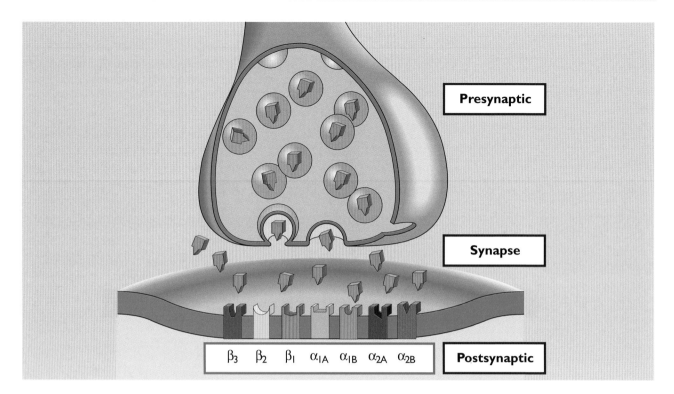

Figure 7.13 The norepinephrine synapse

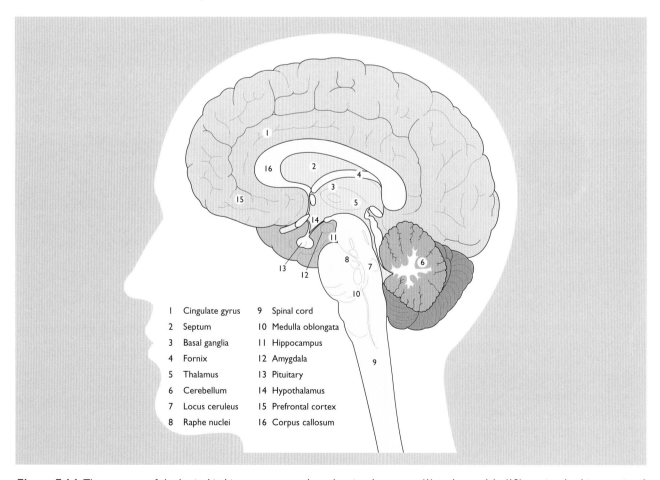

1	Cingulate gyrus	9	Spinal cord
2	Septum	10	Medulla oblongata
3	Basal ganglia	11	Hippocampus
4	Fornix	12	Amygdala
5	Thalamus	13	Pituitary
6	Cerebellum	14	Hypothalamus
7	Locus ceruleus	15	Prefrontal cortex
8	Raphe nuclei	16	Corpus callosum

Figure 7.14 The anatomy of the brain. Limbic structures such as the cingulate gyrus (1) and amygdala (12) are involved in emotional responses, and abnormalities in the function of the system may underpin states of depression

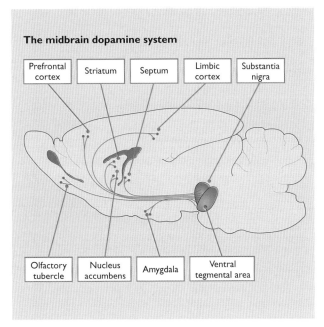

Figure 7.15 The dopaminergic pathways of the rat brain, which are involved in reward mechanisms in animals and in the experience of pleasure in humans

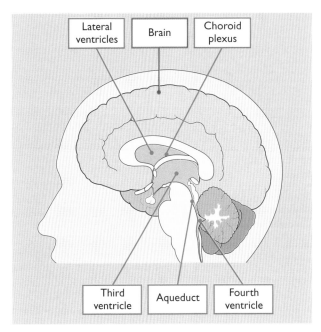

Figure 7.16 Some magnetic resonance imaging and computed tomography studies have shown enlarged lateral and third ventricles in some bipolar patients

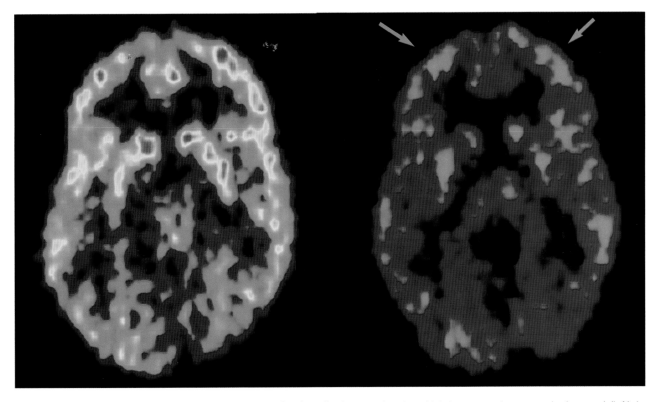

Figure 7.17 Positron emission tomography scanning of a clinically depressed patient (right) compared to a matched control (left). In the color scheme, blue represents less activity (glucose metabolism) while red represents more (glucose metabolism). Note the relative hypoactivity of the cortex on the right with marked hypoactivity of the prefrontal, frontal and deeper basal ganglia that agrees with current theory on the neuropathology of depression. Although some units claim that depression can be shown using imaging techniques, there is no current evidence to suggest that it can be diagnostic in all cases. Reproduced with permission from Dr George. FDG PET Imaging of Depression, http://www.musc.edu/psychiatry/fnrd/petdep.htm

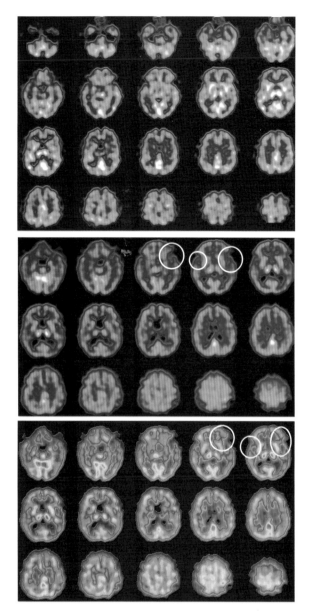

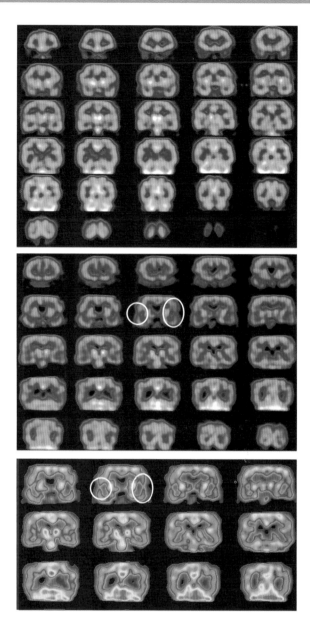

Figure 7.18 HMPAO single-photon emission computed tomography scans (red and green scales) in the transaxial plane of a normal man (top) and an 88-year-old man with clinical depression (middle and bottom). Circled areas represent reduced perfusion to the frontotemporal cortex bilaterally. Printed with permission from the Department of Radiology, Brigham and Women's Hospital, Boston, MA, USA. http://brighamrad.harvard.edu/education/online/BrainSPECT/

Figure 7.19 Single-photon emission computed tomography scans (red and green scales) in the coronal plane of a normal individual (top) and an 88-year-old man with clinical depression (middle and bottom). Circled areas represent reduced perfusion to the frontotemporal cortex bilaterally. Printed with permission from the Department of Radiology, Brigham and Women's Hospital, Boston, MA, USA. http://brighamrad.harvard.edu/education/online/BrainSPECT/

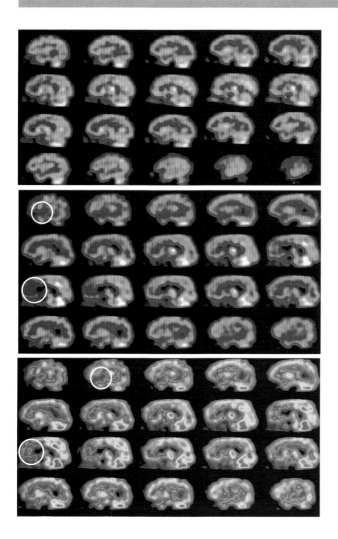

Figure 7.20 Single-photon emission computed tomography scans (red and green scales) in the sagittal plane of a normal individual (top) and an 88-year-old man with clinical depression (middle and bottom). Circled areas represent reduced perfusion to the frontotemporal cortex. Printed with permission from the Department of Radiology, Brigham and Women's Hospital, Boston, MA, USA. http://brighamrad.harvard.edu/education/online/BrainSPECT/

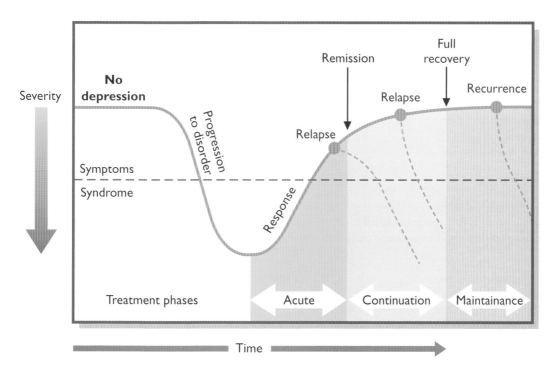

Figure 8.1 Treatment phases in depression. Adapted with permission from Kupfer DJ. Long-term treatment of depression. *J Clin Psychiatry* 1991;52 (suppl):28–34

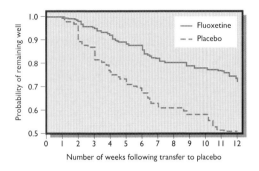

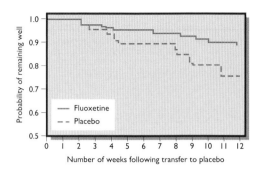

Figure 8.2 Continuation treatment of depression over 3 months. Survival analysis comparing treatment with fluoxetine and placebo during treatment weeks 12 and 24. After 3 months of open-label treatment, continuing with fluoxetine prevents relapse of depressive symptoms in the next 3 months. Adapted with permission from Reimherr FW, Amsterdam HD, Quitkin FM, et al. Optimal length of continuation therapy in depression: a prospective assessment during long-term treatment with fluoxetine. *Am J Psychiatry* 1998;155:1247–53

Figure 8.3 Continuation treatment of depression after 6 months. Survival analysis comparing treatment with fluoxetine and placebo during treatment weeks 26 and 38. After 6 months of treatment, continuing with fluoxetine prevents relapse of depressive symptoms in the next 3 months. Adapted with permission from Reimherr FW, Amsterdam HD, Quitkin FM, et al. Optimal length of continuation therapy in depression: a prospective assessment during long-term treatment with fluoxetine. *Am J Psychiatry* 1998;155:1247–53

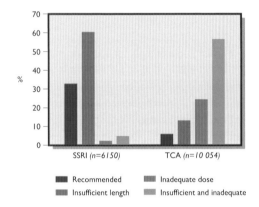

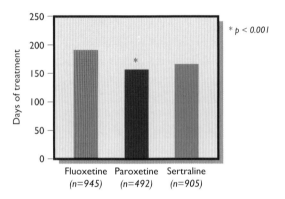

Figure 8.4 Dosage and duration of antidepressant drugs. Adapted with permission from Dunn RL, Donoghue JM, Ozminkowski RJ, et al. Longitudinal patterns of antidepressant prescribing in primary care in the UK: comparison with treatment guidelines. *J Psychopharmacol* 1999;13:136–43. © British Association for Psychopharmacology, 1999)

Figure 8.5 Duration of SSRI treatment. Adapted with permission from Russell JM, Berndt ER, Miceli R, Colucci S, Grudzinski AN. Course and cost of treatment for depression with fluoxetine, paroxetine, and sertraline. *Am J Manag Care* 1999;5:597–606

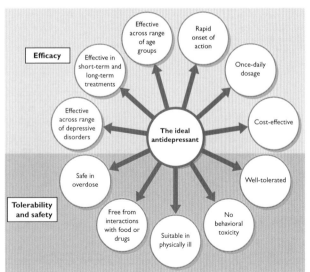

Figure 9.1 The ideal antidepressant

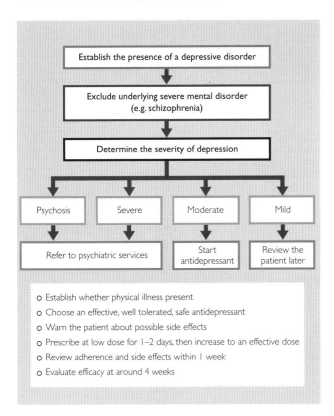

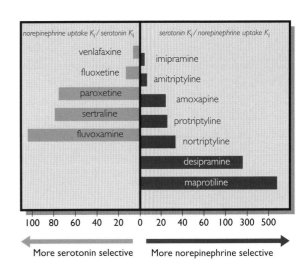

Figure 9.3 Spectrum of action of selected antidepressants

Figure 9.2 Criteria for starting patients on antidepressants

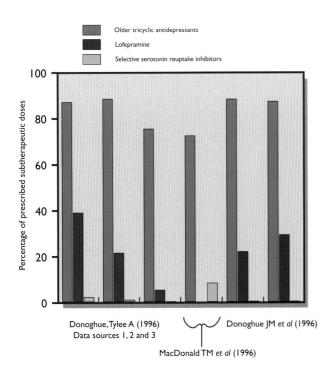

Figure 9.4 Primary care prescribing of antidepressants

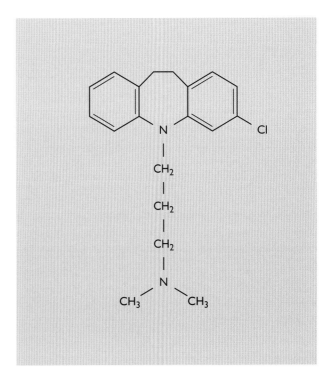

Figure 9.5 Molecular structure of clomipramine, an example of a tricyclic antidepressant

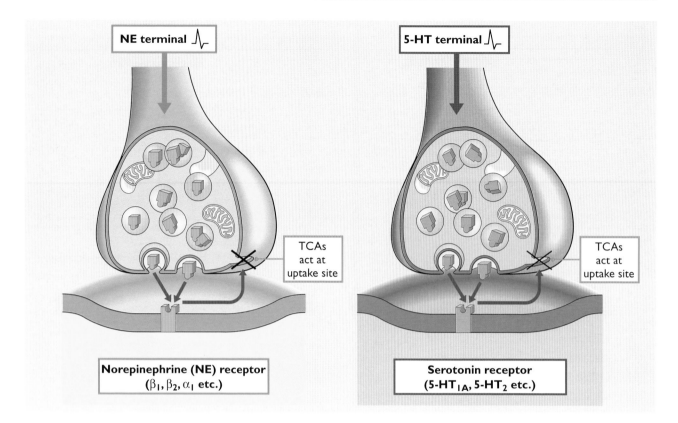

Figure 9.6 Tricyclic antidepressant (TCA) mode of action. TCAs inhibit the reuptake of serotonin and norepinephrine into presynaptic neurones. Additional effects at other receptors (e.g. anticholinergic effects) are largely responsible for adverse effects

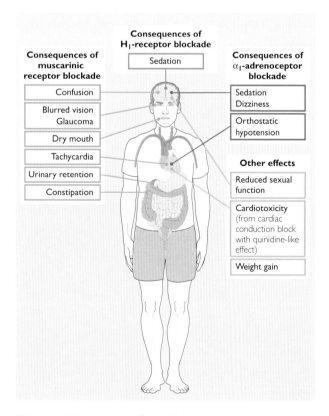

Figure 9.7 Typical side-effects of the tricyclic antidepressants

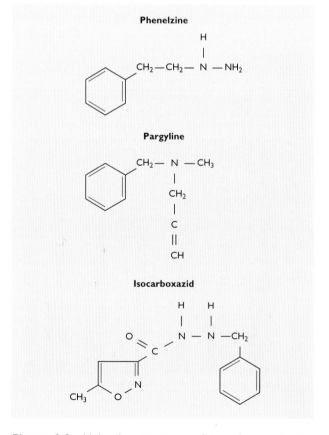

Figure 9.8 Molecular structures of typical non-selective MAOIs (phenelzine, pargyline and isocarboxazid)

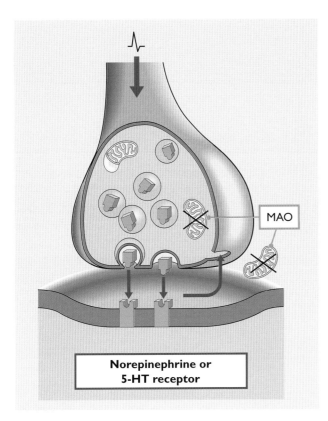

Figure 9.9 MAOI mode of action. MAOI antidepressants inhibit the breakdown of norepinephrine and serotonin, and increase their availability at postsynaptic receptors

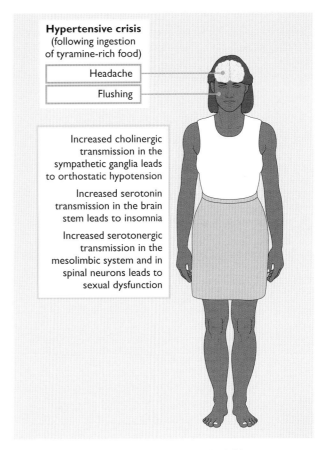

Figure 9.10 The reported side-effects of MAOIs

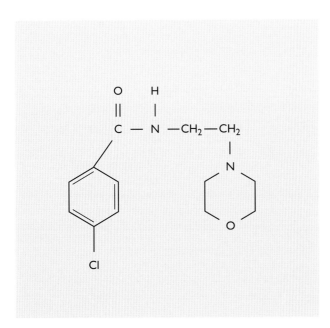

Figure 9.11 The molecular structure of the reversible selective monoamine oxidase inhibitor (MAOI) moclobemide

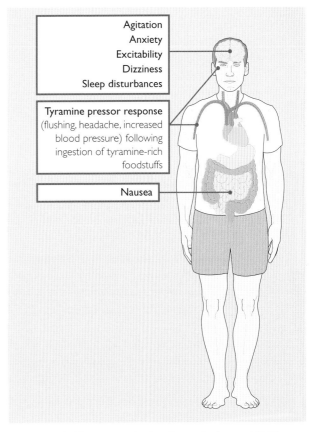

Figure 9.12 The reported side-effects of selective MAOIs

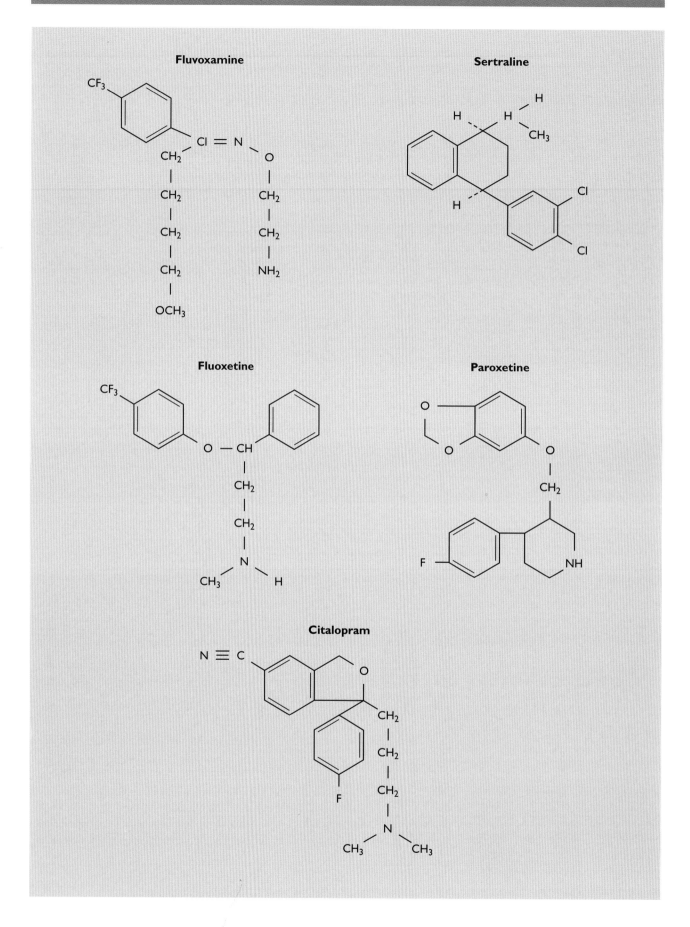

Figure 9.13 Molecular structures for various SSRIs

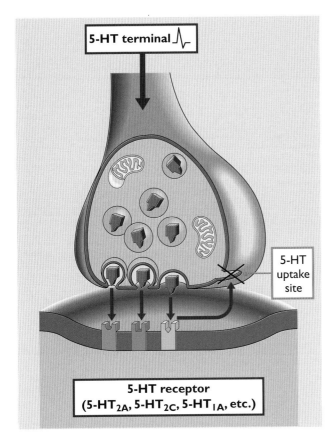

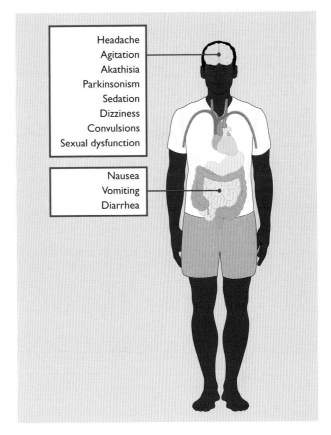

Figure 9.14 SSRI mode of action. SSRIs inhibit reuptake of 5-HT into presynaptic neurones. Increased availability at 5-HT_{1A} receptors is probably responsible for antidepressant efficacy. Actions at other receptors may result in adverse effects: anxiety, insomnia and sexual dysfunction (5-HT_2), and nausea and vomiting (5-HT_3)

Figure 9.15 SSRI side-effects

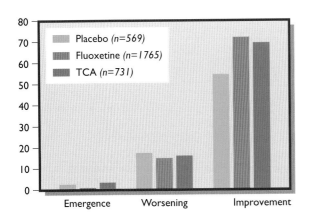

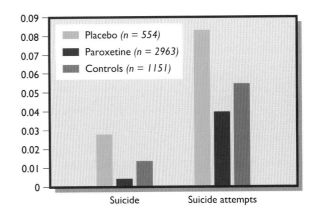

Figure 9.16 SSRIs are not associated with a worsening of suicidal thoughts, as shown by this pooled analysis of 17 randomized controlled trials using suicide item of HAM-D. Adapted with permission from Beasley CM, Dornseif BE, Bosomworth JC, et al. Fluoxetine and suicide: a meta-analysis of controlled trials of treatment for depression. Br Med J 1991;303:685–92

Figure 9.17 A pooled analysis of randomized controlled trials of paroxetine showing it is not associated with an increase in suicidal behavior. Adapted from Eur Neuropsychopharmacol 1995;5:5–13. Montgomery SA, Dunner DL, Dunbar GC. Reduction of suicidal thoughts with paroxetine in comparison with reference antidepressants and placebo. PEY, patient-exposure years. Copyright 1995, with permission from Elsevier Science

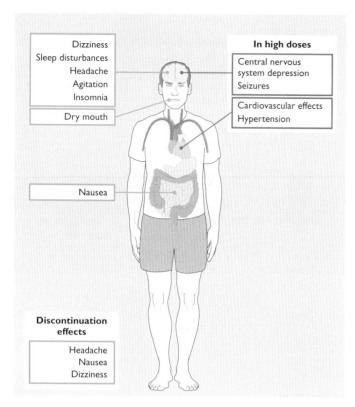

Figure 9.18 Molecular structures of SNRIs venlafaxine and milnacipran

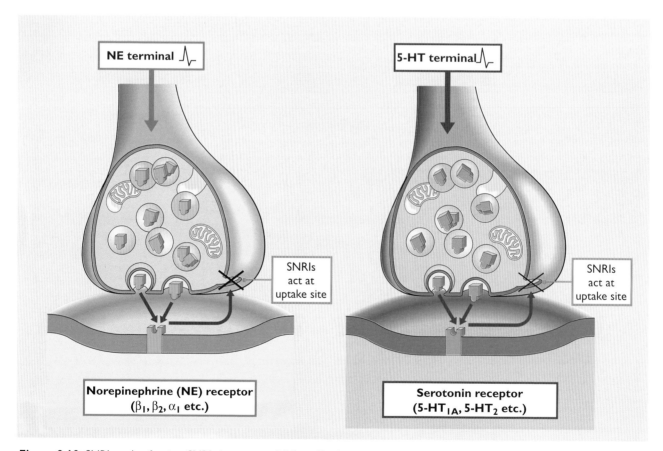

Figure 9.19 SNRI mode of action. SNRIs increase availability of both serotonin and norepinephrine without unwanted interactions at postsynaptic receptors

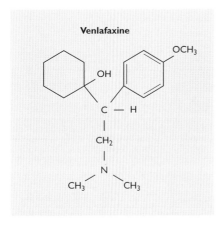

Venlafaxine

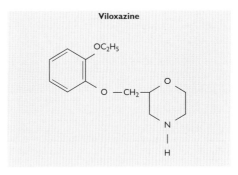

Viloxazine

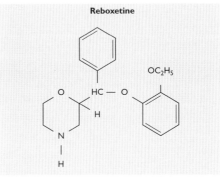

Reboxetine

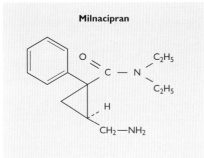

Milnacipran

Figure 9.20 Side-effects seen with SNRIs

Figure 9.21 Examples of norepinephrine reuptake inhibitors. Reboxetine is now termed a selective norepinephrine reuptake inhibitor

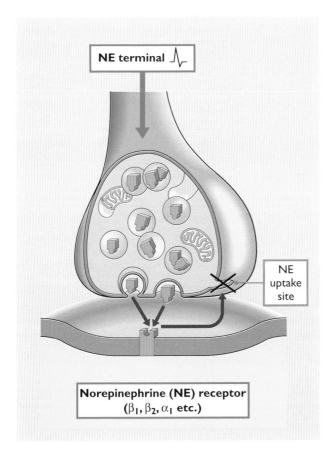

Figure 9.22 Mode of action of norepinephrine inhibitors. Increase availability of norepinephrine may result in improved mood, drive and capacity for social interaction

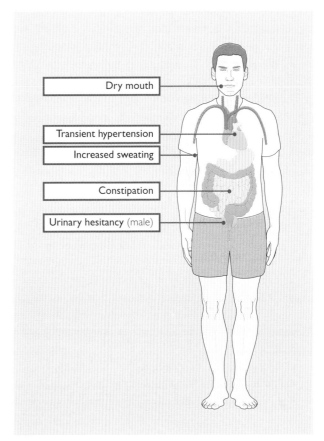

Figure 9.23 Side-effects of norepinephrine reuptake inhibitors

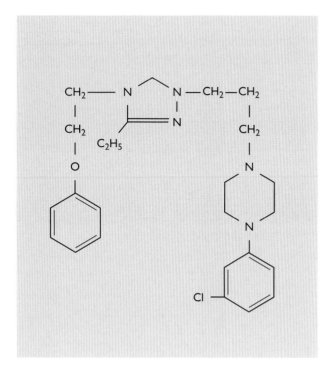

Figure 9.24 Molecular structure of nefazodone

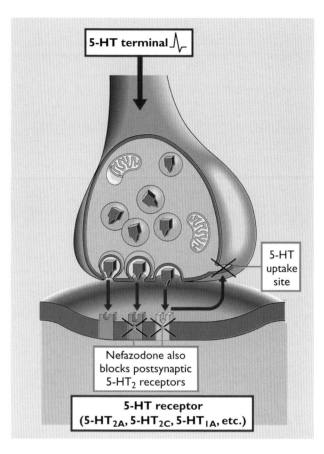

Figure 9.25 The mode of action of nefazodone. Similar to the mode of action of SSRIs, nefazodone blocks 5-HT reuptake, but in addition blocks postsynaptic 5-HT₂ receptors

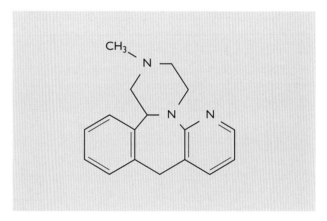

Figure 9.27 Molecular structure of mirtazapine

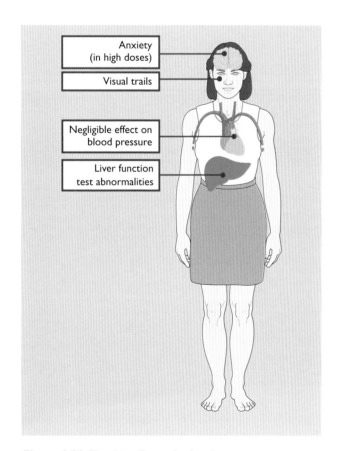

Figure 9.26 The side-effects of nefazodone

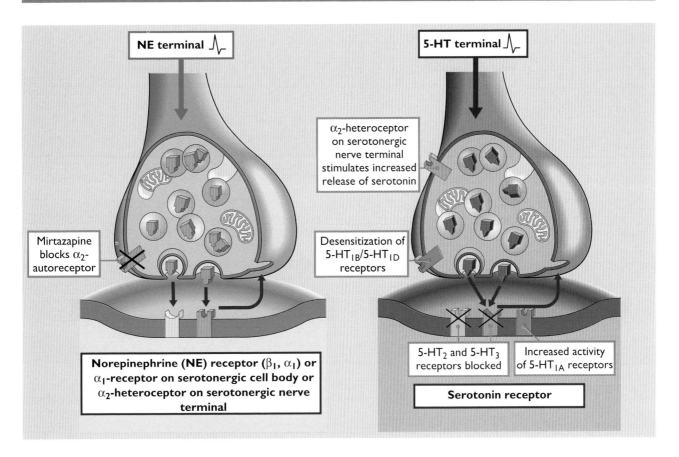

Figure 9.28 The mode of action of mirtazapine. Mirtazapine enhances noradrenergic and serotonergic function by blocking the inhibitory α_2-adrenoceptors on noradrenergic terminals and the α_2-heteroceptors on serotonergic terminals

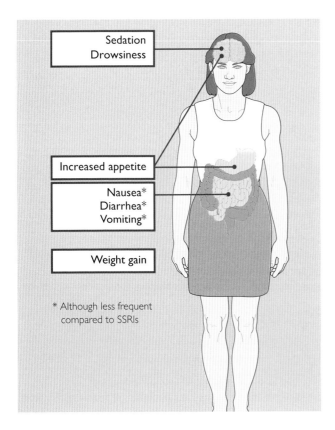

Figure 9.29 The side-effects of mirtazapine

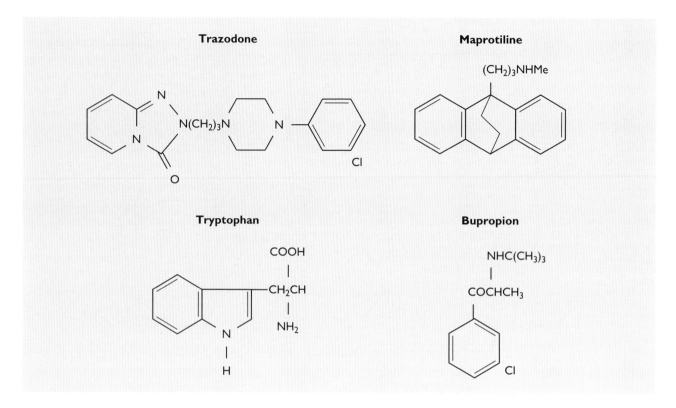

Figure 9.30 Molecular structures of trazodone, maprotiline, L-tryptophan and bupropion

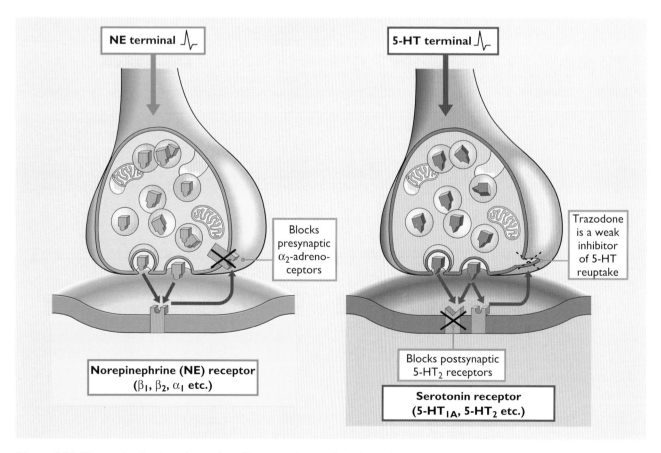

Figure 9.31 The mode of action of trazodone. Trazodone is a weak inhibitor of serotonin reuptake and can increase norepinephrine release as a result of its antagonistic action on presynaptic α_2-adrenoceptors. It also blocks postsynaptic 5-HT$_2$ receptors

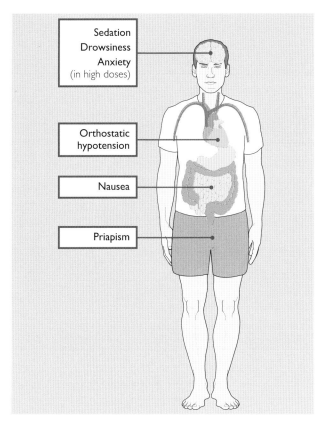

Figure 9.32 Side-effects of trazodone

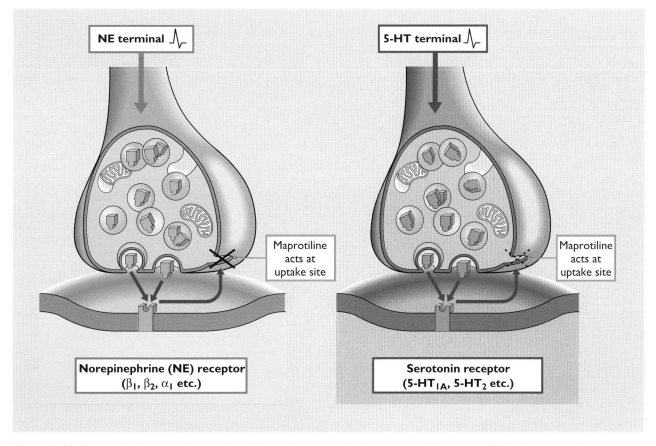

Figure 9.33 The mode of action of maprotiline. Maprotiline is a modified tricyclic antidepresssant (TCA) that has similar efficacy to the TCAs

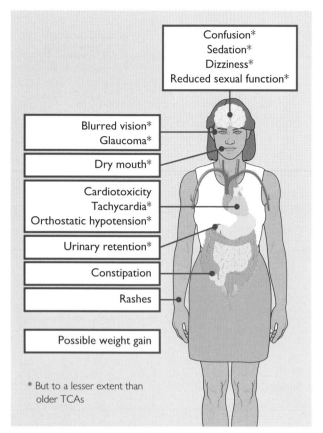

Figure 9.34 The side-effects of maprotiline

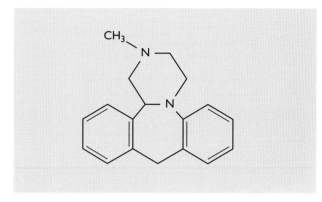

Figure 9.35 Molecular structure of mianserin

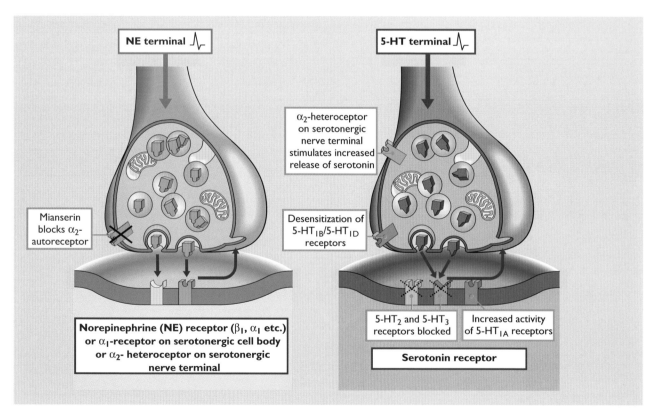

Figure 9.36 The mode of action of mianserin. Mianserin, like mirtazapine, enhances noradrenergic and serotonergic function by blocking the inhibitory α_2-adrenoceptors on noradrenergic terminals and the α_2-heteroceptors on serotonergic terminals. However, mirtazapine is more effective than mianserin in enhancing serotonergic function, as it increases the firing rate of serotonergic neurons. Mianserin is less potent in blocking postsynaptic serotonin receptors

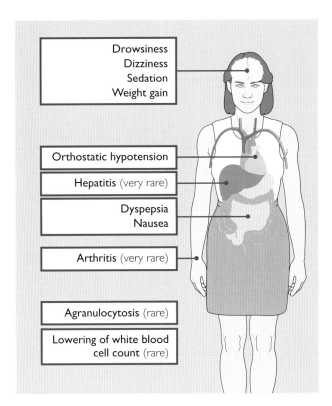

Figure 9.37 The side-effects of mianserin

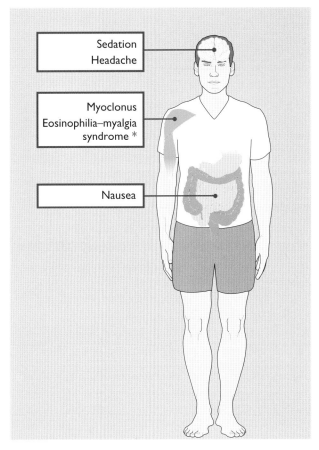

Figure 9.38 The side-effects of L-tryptophan. *, Eosinophilia–myalgia syndrome was linked to contamination of some tryptophan-containing products during the manufacturing process, therefore close monitoring is required

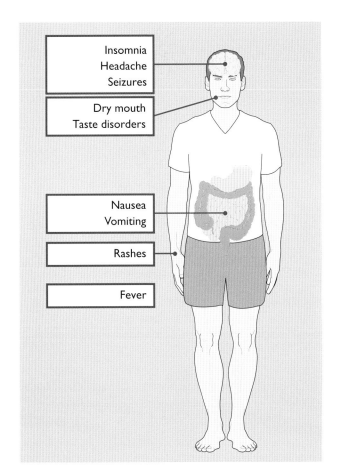

Figure 9.39 The side-effects of bupropion

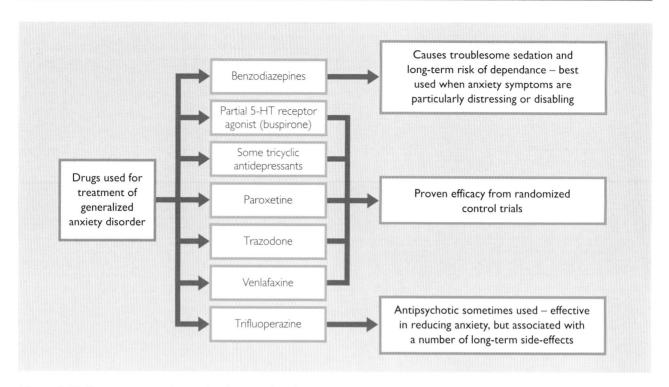

Figure 9.40 Drug treatment of generalized anxiety disorder

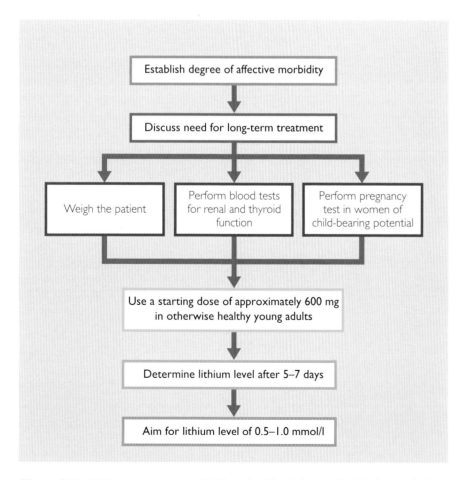

Figure 9.41 Lithium treatment plan. Lithium should only be used in bipolar prophylaxis when it is reasonable to anticipate treatment lasting more than 2 years. Shorter periods of treatment are associated with an increased risk of rebound mania on stopping lithium

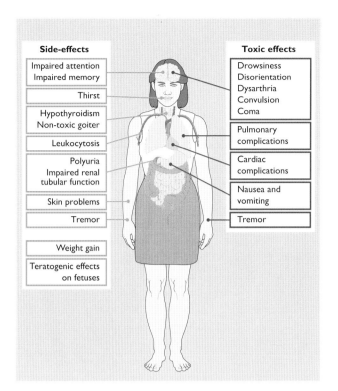

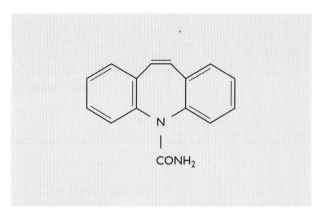

Figure 9.43 Example of an anticonvulsant drug (carbamazepine). Carbemazepine has the tricyclic structure of many older antidepressants and conventional antipsychotic drugs

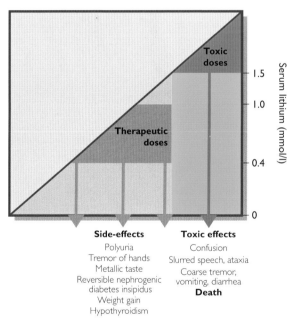

Figure 9.42 The side-effects of lithium and its spectrum of action. Graph reproduced with permission from Stevens L, Rodn I. *Psychiatry: an Illustrated Colour Text.* Edinburgh: Churchill Livingstone, 2001:25

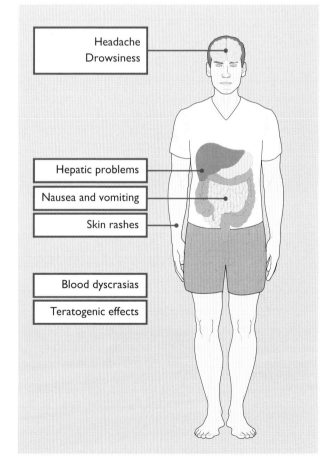

Figure 9.44 The general side-effects of anticonvulsants. However, drugs differ in their relative propensity to cause particular adverse effects. Always refer to the prescribers information

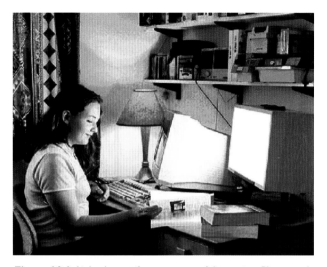

Figure 10.1 Light therapy for treatment of depression. Photograph courtesy of SAD Lightbox Co. Ltd., High Wycombe, UK

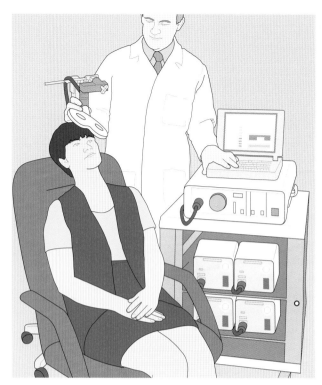

Figure 10.2 Transcranial magnetic stimulation is stil an experimental approach to the treatment of depression. It appears to show efficacy in acute treatment and may have value in continuation treatment

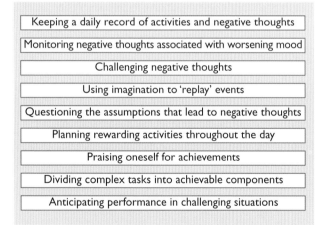

Figure 11.1 The techniques of cognitive–behavior therapy

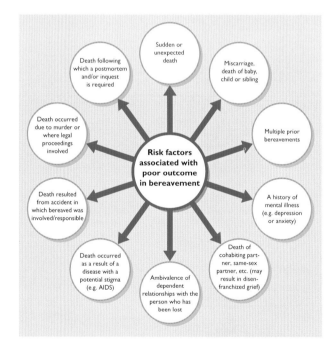

Figure 11.2 Risk factors associated with bereavement

Index

U
unipolar depression 17
urinary hesitancy 45

V
valproate 51, 52
venlafaxine 44, 108, 109
  adverse effects/interactions 41, 44
  in anxiety disorders 49, 50
ventricle–brain ratio 34, 99
viloxazine 109
vulnerability factors 35

W
widowed patients 20–1, 30
'winter blues' 19

Z
'Zurich criteria', recurrent brief depression 19, 78